Schistosomiasis of Animals in Uzbekistan

Authored by Djalaliddin Azimov

Published in London, United Kingdom

Schistosomiasis of Animals in Uzbekistan
http://dx.doi.org/10.5772/intechopen.109826
Edited by Djalaliddin Azimov

Contributors
Djalaliddin A. Azimov, Bakhrom T. Norkobilov, Erkin B. Shakarboev, Alisher A. Safarov, Ulugbek A. Shakarbaev, Firuza D. Akramova

First published in London, United Kingdom, 2026 by IntechOpen
IntechOpen is the global imprint of INTECHOPEN LIMITED, registered in England and Wales, registration number: 11086078, 167-169 Great Portland Street, London, W1W 5PF, United Kingdom

For EU product safety concerns: IN TECH d.o.o., Prolaz Marije Krucifikse Kozulić 3, 51000 Rijeka, Croatia, info@intechopen.com or visit our website at intechopen.com.

British Library Cataloguing-in-Publication Data
A catalogue record for this book is available from the British Library

Schistosomiasis of Animals in Uzbekistan
Edited by Djalaliddin Azimov
p. cm.
Print ISBN 978-1-80632-105-6
Online ISBN 978-1-80632-104-9
eBook (PDF) ISBN 978-1-80632-106-3

Meet the editor

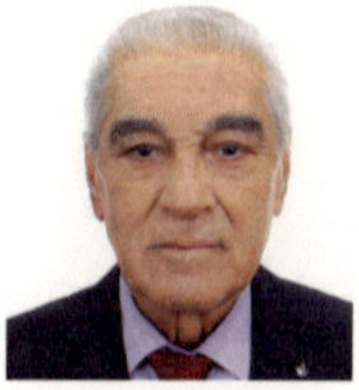

Dr. Azimov Djalaliddin Azimovich, DSc, is an academician of the Academy of Sciences of the Republic of Uzbekistan; chief researcher of the Laboratory of General Parasitology, Institute of Zoology, Academy of Sciences of the Republic of Uzbekistan; professor in the Department of Zoology, National University of Uzbekistan; consultant for the Committee for Veterinary and Livestock Development of the Republic of Uzbekistan and member of the Governing Council, Samarkand State University of Veterinary Medicine, Livestock and Biotechnology. He is a member, scientific advisor, and regional expert of international organizations and conventions, including the International Union for Conservation of Nature (IUCN), the World Wildlife Fund (WWF), the Convention on the Conservation of Migratory Species of Wild Animals (CMS), and the Convention on Biological Diversity (CBD). Dr. Djaloliddin Azimov is a specialist in general and veterinary parasitology. His research interests include problems in population biology and ecology, phylogeny, evolution, schistosome taxonomy, and mechanisms of host–parasite interactions. He is the author of more than 1000 papers on biodiversity conservation and general and veterinary parasitology.

Contents

Preface

Although there is already extensive literature on schistosomatids and schistosomiasis in animals and humans, we are unaware of any publications devoted explicitly to schistosomiasis caused by the trematode *Schistosoma turkestanicum* Skrjabin, 1913.

Schistosomiasis of Animals in Uzbekistan has no English-language analogues, but this does not mean that similar work has not been carried out worldwide. Such work has been conducted for decades in many countries of Asia, Europe, and Africa by thousands of researchers, zoologists, parasitologists, veterinarians, teachers, students, and naturalists. There may be extensive information available on *Sch. turkestanicum*, a widespread trematode of agricultural and wild commercial mammals across many geographical areas of the world. Unfortunately, it has not been compiled or generalized by anyone. There is a lot of information available on the organism's biology, life cycle, and distribution among animals in many countries of Europe and Asia, and this work is an attempt to systematize this information and compare and contrast it with what has been studied and found in Uzbekistan specifically.

The authors of the book consider the problems of animal schistosomiasis from two perspectives. On the one hand, *Sch. turkestanicum* is the causative agent of serious helminthiasis in both domestic and wild animals. This is the reason for the rapid development of applied trematodology, which has a pronounced veterinary and medical-sanitary character. On the other hand, schistosomes, with their unique life cycle, have become the object of general zoological and parasitological research.

This book discusses fundamental and applied problems of schistosomiasis, a parasitic disease caused by *Sch. turkestanicum* ("blood flukes"), which parasitizes as adults in the circulatory systems of several mammalian species and at the miracidia and sporocyst stages in aquatic mollusks of various species of the genus *Lymnaea* (= Radix) Cercariae. Emerging from infected mollusks, they live in water as free-swimming adults for a short time and, to continue development, must infect the circulatory system of the final host and form dioecious schistosomes. Cercariae are the invasive stage, which is dangerous for mammals. Schistosomiasis is widespread worldwide, primarily in tropical and temperate regions. Outbreaks of schistosomiasis have occurred in many countries and cause significant damage to livestock sectors.

With this book, we aim to satisfy the interests of a wide range of readers, from those engaged in the practical fight against schistosomiasis to general parasitologists seeking information. Readers interested in the issues raised here in a more general form are directed to the introductory and concluding chapters. These chapters cover not only current achievements and future prospects but also research and development proposals for those responsible for planning and funding future work. For the convenience of most specialist readers, all material is divided into separate topics, some of which are more general, while others are more narrowly specialized. The book also incorporates studies yet to be published to provide a look into the future. We hope this book will prove to be a useful guide for general biologists, zoologists, and parasitologists and will serve as a catalyst, accelerating further research in the field.

Djalaliddin A. Azimov
Laboratory of General Parasitology,
Institute of Zoology of the Academy of Sciences of the Republic of Uzbekistan,
Tashkent, Uzbekistan

Foreword

One of the most important scientific directions of the Institute of Zoology Academy of Sciences of the Republic of Uzbekistan is the preparation of big monographs, dedicated to the problems of general parasitology, which are to have medical and veterinary significants.

This book is the authors' first monographic research on schistosomiasis, one of the most dangerous animal diseases. This disease is distributed in some Asian and European states; it is recorded in two epizootological forms: synanthropic, the concentrations of which are present in many regions with developed animal breeding and natural—in wild animals.

Since the 1980s until recently, significant success has been achieved in the study of this disease, especially in the clarification of its epizootology and the exploration of specific methods and ways of its treatment. Significant achievements in understanding this problem are connected with the authors of this monograph under the guidance of Academician D.A. Azimov. The results of long-term studies on this problem are known not only in Uzbekistan, but also in many other countries of the world.

The main issues of pathogen biology, epizootology, pathogenesis, pathohistology,diagnosis and treatment of animal schistosomiasis, as well as aspects of the epidemiology of human cercarioses are discussed in the book.

In conclusion, it should be noted that a deep analysis and professional generalisationof literature data and inclusion of materials from the huge experimental work enabled the authors of this monograph to create an interesting work full of factual materials, which will no doubt solve successfully the transcontinental problem—schistosomiasis of animals caused by Schistosoma turkestanicum Skrjabin, 1913.

Djalaliddin A. Azimov

Dedicated to the Bright Memory—Great Scientist, Founder of the Helminthologists School, Academician, Konstantin Ivanovich Skrjabin

Chapter 1

Introduction

Djalaliddin A. Azimov

Schistosomiasis of humans and animals is one of the most important parasitic diseases of the parasitic diseases of human and animals from the social and economic aspects.

The schistosomiasis caused by *Schistosoma turkestanicum*, is reported for the first time as a disease of the domestic animals of Iraq in 1936 [1]. The researcher examined the life cycle of this trematode and established its intermediate host, which was mollusc Lymnaea tenera euphratica. The author reported that up to 80% of sheep, goats and cattle, including buffalo, and about 15% of horses, mules, donkeys and camels in the wetlands of Iraq, near rice plantations on both sides of the Tigris, were infected with this parasite.

MacHattie's work drew the attention of parasitologists, which resulted in other reports from both Iraq and other Asian and European countries about *Sch. turkestanicum* found in different animals. Between 1936 and 1966 Schistosoma was found in the mammals of Iraq, Iran, Pakistan, India, China, Azerbaijan, Kazakhstan, Kyrgyzstan, Turkmenistan, Russia, Uzbekistan and France [2].

In 1965, 1985 and 2005, three major outbreaks of schistosomiasis were recorded in the Republic of Karakalpakstan and Khorezm Province (both in Uzbekistan) infecting hundreds of thousands of sheep and cattle, over 50% of which died, the rest having been euthanised, as at that time there were no effective remedies. As the epizootic situation was so grave that active research into the biology, ecology, epizootology, pathogenesis, diagnostics, treatment and prevention of schistosomiasis of animals was launched [3].

Although scientists have achieved good results in studying the problem of schistosomiasis of animals, in most countries this disease remains highly infectious. For instance, until recently schistosomiasis was recorded only in the farms of the lower course of the Amudarya (Republic of Karakalpakstan and Khorezm Province in Uzbekistan and Dashoguz Province in Turkmenistan), and now within Uzbekistan, the domestic animals from the lower course of the Syrdarya River (Tashkent and Syrdarya Provinces) are reported to be infected with this disease [3]. Other Asian and European countries also reported about a wide distribution of *Sch. turkestanicum* [4–13] confirm that the parasite causing schistosomiasis is widely distributed in the abovementioned regions. It should be noted that the latest report about *Sch. turkestanicum* was recorded in the European red deer in Hungary in 2010.

Currently, the epizootic situation connected with *Sch. turkestanicum* in Uzbekistan remains grave, which requires constant monitoring of the animals and taking preventive measures. In addition, the medicinal aspects of schistosomiasis in the infection regions have been established. The cercariae of this trematode cause non-specific cercarioses [14–17].

As cases of human cercarioses have become more frequent, the research into the problem is becoming increasingly active throughout the area they are spread around [9, 13, 18–20]. Cercarioses of humans caused by the cercariae *Sch. turkestanicum* have been recorded in many European and Asian countries.

Populations of *Schistosoma turkestanicum* are widely distributed in aquatic and semi-aquatic ecosystems—the principal habitats of wild and domestic animals. They live in the blood vessels of mammals causing serious diseases in animals and great damage to cattle breeding. Scientists have discovered complex relations between the parasite and host, which can be detected in the morphologic and functional deviations of the organs and systems leading to a considerable decrease of cattle's productivity [3].

The disease seems to have become a serious transcontinental veterinary and medical problem at present.

All these problems associated with schistosomiasis have become the subject of this monograph. The data throughout the monograph are based on the research carried out between 1965 and 2014, including the work done at different farms in the Republic of Karakalpakstan and Khorezm, Tashkent and Syrdarya Provinces of Uzbekistan. This information is interesting from all biological aspects and would be of use for researchers and specialists in the veterinary and medical sciences.

We think it is our duty to dedicate this chapter in the memory of academician K.I. Skrjabin, the founder of the school of helminthology in the territory of the former USSR. He initiated this research and was very interested in and concerned about till his last days.

We are deeply grateful to the staff of the laboratory for general parasitology at the Institute of Zoology under the Academy of Sciences of the Republic of Uzbekistan for their practical support in the course of the research. We are very thankful to the experts from the veterinary service of the Republic of Karakalpakstan, who assisted us considerably in our field and experimental work.

Acknowledgements

We would also love to thank our colleagues from abroad—doctors A.S. Chauhan, C.B. Srivastava, B.S. Chauhan V. Kumar, J. Massoud, B.P. Singh and R.P. Mukerjee, who provided us with their interesting works on trematodes from the genus schistosoma.

Conflicts of interest

The authors declare no conflict of interest.

Author details

Djalaliddin A. Azimov
Institute of Zoology of the Academy of Sciences of the Republic of Uzbekistan, Tashkent, Uzbekistan

*Address all correspondence to: safarov-alisher@mail.ru

References

[1] Machattie C. A preliminary note on the life history of Schistosoma turkestanicum Skrjabin, 1913. Transactions of the Royal Society of Tropical Medicine and Hygiene. 1936;**30**:115-124

[2] Azimov DA. The Schistosomes of Animals and Humans. Tashkent: Fan; 1975. p. 152

[3] Azimov DA. Tremadodes—Parasites of Animals and Human. Tashkent: Mehnat; 1986. p. 128

[4] Kumar V. Studies on snail hosts of Orientobilharzia turkestanicum (Skrjabin, 1913) Dutt et Srivastava, 1955 (Schistosomatidae: Trematoda) in India. Annales de la Societe belge de medecine tropicale. 1973;**53**(1):17-23

[5] Massoud J. Studies on the Schistosomes of domestic animals in Iran. I. Observations on Ornithobilharzia turkestanica (Skrjabin, 1913) in Khuzestan. Journal of Helminthology. 1973;**67**(2):165-180

[6] Chauhan AS, Srivastava CB, Chauhan BS. Studies on the trematode fauna of India. Part 6. Digenea: Schistosomatidae. A monographie aid to the identification of Indian schistosomes. Journal of the Zoological Society of India. 1973;**25**(12):83-127

[7] Chien-an L, Kung-mao P, Lung S, Chao-ming L, Min-sen C, Chung L. A survey of the aetiological agent of rice-field dermatitis in Chegnan peoples commune, Hailung Hsien, Kirin Province, with a preliminary observation of the life history of Orientobilharzia turkestanica var. tuberculata. Dunu syuabao, Acta Zoologica Sinica. 1975;**21**(2):183-189

[8] Tang C, Tang Z, Cao H, Tang L, Yu CQQ, Lu H. Research into Orientobilharzia turkestanica parasitizing sheep in the eastern part of an autonomous district in Inner Mongolia. Dunu syuebao, Acta Zoologica Sinica. 1983;**29**(3):249-255

[9] Wang CR, Han Y, Xu LM, Yu WC, Qiu JH, Yu KJ, et al. Observation of effect of "Kangxuexichong II" against Orientobilharzia spp. In naturally infective sheep. Journal of Animal Science and Veterinary Medicine. 2000;**6**:20-21

[10] Lockyer AE, Olson PD, Littlewood DTJ. Utility of complete large and small subunit rRNA genes in resolving the phylogeny of the Platyhelminthes: Implications and review of the cercomer theory. Biologikal Journal of the Linnean Society. 2003;**78**:155-173

[11] Li L, Yu LY, Zhu XQ, Wang CR, Zhai YQ, Zhao JP. Orientobilharzia turkestanicum is grouped within African schistosomes based on phylogenetic analyses using sequences of mitochondrial genes. Parasitology Research. 2008;**102**:939-943

[12] Qiu JH, Li L, Wang CR, Chen J, Chen AH, Zhai YQ. ITS and 28S rDNA-LSU sequence analysis of Orientobilharzia turkestanicum from bovine and caprine hosts. Chinese Journal of Parasitology. 2008;**26**(3):183

[13] Majoros G, Dán A, Erdélyi K. A natural focus of the blood fluke *Orientobilharzia turkestanica* (Skrjabin, 1913) (Trematoda: Schistosomatidae) in red deer (Cervus elaphus) in Hungery. Veterinary Parasitology. 2010;**170**(3-4):218-223

[14] Azimov DA, Arifjanov ZK. Research into the blood serum proteins of sheep infected experimentally with orientobilharziasis. In: The Works of all-Russian K.I. Skrjabin Scientific Research Institute of Helmonthology. Vol. 15. Moscow: Nauka; 1969. pp. 25-32

[15] Azimov DA, Shakarboev EB, Isakova DT, Akramova FD. Annotated Dictionary of Parasitology Terms. Tashkent: Fan; 2007. p. 210

[16] Shakarboyev EB. Trematodes of the Vertebrates of Uzbekistan (the Species Composition, Circulation Ways, Ecology Ad Biology): A Doctoral Thesis in Biology. Tashkent: Institute of Zoology; 2009. p. 243

[17] Azimov DA, Akramova FD, Shakarbayev UA, Shakarboyev EB. Orientobildgarsii—Mammalian Trematodes. Tashkent: Fan; 2014. p. 224

[18] Sahba Gholam HA, Malek EA. Dermatitis caused by cercariae of Orientobilharzia turkestanica in the Caspian Sea area of Iran. American Journal of Tropical Medicine and Hygiene. 1979;**28**(5):912-912

[19] Athari A, Amini H, Sahba GH. Investigation of cercarial dermatitis in Iran. Bulletin de la Societe Française de Parasitologie. 1990;**8**(Suppl 2):888

[20] Amid A, Gohar S, Rosnami M. Dermination of definitive and intermediate hosts of cercarial dermatitis-producing agents in northern Iran. Archives of Iranian Medicine. 2006;**9**(1):11-15

Chapter 2

The History of the Transformation of Knowledge about *Schistosoma Turkestanicum*, Parasite of Animals

Djalaliddin A. Azimov, Firuza D. Akramova and Ulugbek A. Shakarbaev

Abstract

This chapter presents information about the findings of four species of the genus *Schistosoma* Weinland, 1858; *Schistosoma bomfordi* Montgomeri, 1906; *Schistosoma turkestanicum* Skrjabin, 1913, *Schistosoma dattai* (Dutt et Srivastava, 1955), and *Schistosoma harinasutai* (Kruatrachue, Bhaibulaja, Harinasuta, 1965)—animal parasites. These schistosomes are common in many countries of Asia and Europe. More than 20 species of mammals, mainly ungulates, have been registered as definitive hosts. Much attention is paid to the widespread type of *Sch. turkestanicum*, on various issues of biology, ecology, pathology and measures of control and prevention of invasion.

Keywords: history, transformation, *Schistosoma turkestanicum*, *Sch. bomfordi*, *Sch. dattai*, *Sch. harinasutai*, Asia, Europe, Uzbekistan

1. Introduction

The first pieces of information about the trematodes living in blood, which are currently included in the genus *Schistosoma*, were obtained in 1906 when a new species was described and found in the cattle and zebu of India named *Schistosoma bomfordi* Montgomery 1906 (Montgomery, 1906). This species was found in sheep in Russia by R.S. Schultz and S.K. Skrjabin (1928: cit. according to K.I. Skrjabin, 1951)

In 1909 K.I. Skrjabin described the second species, *Schistosoma turkestanicum* Skrjabin, 1913, which he discovered in cattle in Kazakhstan [1]. In the following years two more species from this group, *Schistosoma dattai* and *Sch. harinasutai*, respectively, were discovered in India and Thailand.

Until recently the abovementioned four species of *Schistosoma* [2–7] were transferred from one genus to another and were objects of debate.

The phylogenetic research into the family Schistosomatidae based on molecular markers [8–12] enabled Aldhoun, Littlewood (2012) to make a final specification of the places of the trematodes under study in the genus *Schistosoma* Weinland, 1858. We agree with this viewpoint.

According to the universal opinion, trematodes *Sch. bomfordi, Sch. dattai, Sch. harinasutai* and *Sch. turkestanicum* are included in the genus *Schistosoma* alongside other well-known species. Some populations of the four *Schistosoma* species noted above have been recorded in many countries across Asia and some European countries [7, 12–14].

Thus, currently, the genus *Schistosoma* consists of around 20 species parasitising humans and animals.

In their works Azimov (1965–1993) and Azimov et al. (1967–2014) discuss a range of issues associated with *Schistosoma turkestanicum*. The results of their research have been published widely and specialists are acquainted with them.

Within the habitat of trematode *Schistosoma turkestanicum* about 20 species of mammals (sheep, goats, cattle, buffaloes, zebu, Bactrian and Arabian camels, saiga antelopes, roe deer, elks, deer, horses, donkeys, mules, wild boars, cats and rats) belonging to seven families – Felidae, Muridae, Equidae, Suidae, Cervidae, Bovidae and Camelidae [4, 6, 11–13, 15–30] were recorded to be their definitive hosts.

Six species of freshwater mollusk *Lymnaea* (=*Radix*): *L. tenera, L. peregra, L. auricularia, L. gedroziana*, *L. ovate* and *L. acuminata* [4, 14, 16, 17, 19, 21, 23, 24, 31–37] were recorded as the intermediate hosts of trematodes.

Populations of the species from this genus are associated with certain territories within their habitats, where they form isolated focuses of infection.

The distribution of infections among animals both in Uzbekistan and other countries depends on the distribution of their intermediate hosts—freshwater molluscs from the genius *Lymnaea,* mostly *L. auricularia* [38].

K.K. Uvaliyeva et al. (1968) note that in the southern regions of Kazakhstan, schistosoma uses two species as intermediate hosts—*L. auricularia* and *L. peregra*. The average rate of infection with cercariae in *L. peregra* is 5.19%. The researchers inspected 180 bodies of water in the southern and southeastern parts of Kazakhstan, where they collected 400 specimens of molluscs, among which there were specific species involved in the transmission of *Sch. turkestanicum* to domestic ungulates [39].

Ya.N. Zakhryalov (1971, 1975) reports on the ecology of *L. auricularia plicatula*, schistosoma's intermediate host in the Far East. In the course of the research, he established that the wide distribution of this mollusc over the continental part of the Far East is conditioned by this pond snail's high adaptability to a different environment, allowing it to inhabit water bodies of various types (except for mountain streams with rocky bottoms) with highly diverse chemical and physical characteristics and to enter the winter period in an adult stage, as well as by the mollusc's prolificacy, resulting in its high concentration in the habitats with a maximum in August and September. The rate of infection with *Schistosoma* larvae in this pond snail ranges from 1.1 to 13.1%, depending on its number.

The research carried out by D.F. Stepanov (1969a) showed the role of molluscs in the spreading of schistosomiasis in the productive livestock of Turkmenistan.

Researchers from other countries also noted the role of molluscs from the genus *Lymnaea* in the distribution of *Sch. turkestanicum* in India, Pakistan, Iran and Iraq [4, 16, 17, 19, 21, 22].

Analysis of the indicated materials prove the important role of molluscs from the genus Lymnaea play in the distribution of the studied schistosoma in certain animals in different parts of the world. These pond snails are quite common for the biocoenoses of certain bodies of water. The infected molluscs discharge large numbers of cercariae and spread them, thus, playing an important part in the epizootology of schistosomiasis in productive livestock in the centres of infection.

The information on this aspect of *Sch. turkestanicum* varies in character, reflecting the extent that the problem is studied in different parts of Asia and Europe.

2. The Republic of Uzbekistan

Within Uzbekistan, these trematodes were recorded in the animals of the Republic of Karakalpakstan and in Khorezm, Syrdarya and Tashkent Provinces [7, 40–49].

Infected animals were found in many parts of the country (**Figure 1**).

The northeastern part of Uzbekistan comprises three major provinces: Syrdarya, Tashkent and Jizzakh Provinces. In the first two provinces, schistosoma was recorded in sheep and cattle.

No any schistosoma was detected in the animals of the eastern (Andizhan, Namangan and Fergana Provinces), central (Samarkand, Bukhara and Navoi Provinces) and southern Uzbekistan (Surkhandarya and Kashkadarya Provinces).

The Republic of Karakalpakstan and Khorezm Province lie in the lower course of the Amudarya River, in the northwestern part of Uzbekistan. This is the largest region of Uzbekistan occupying about 42% of its area. In this region, schistosomias is caused by *Sch. turkestanicum* and has a stationary character [7, 50, 51].

3. The Republic of Kyrgyzstan

M.G. Toktouchikova (1971) detected *Sch. turkestanicum* in the cattle of the Issyk Kul depression, with an infection rate of 1.3% and the number of specimens in each animal ranging from 14 to 400.

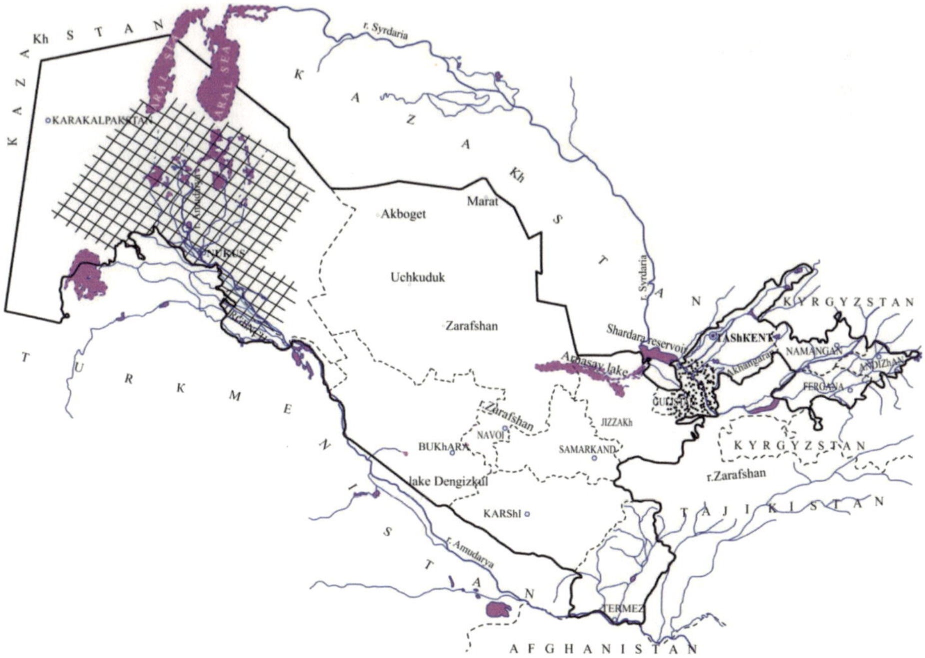

Figure 1.
The distribution areas of trematode Sch. turkestanicum in Uzbekistan: stationary concentration areas; new concentration areas.

4. The Republic of Turkmenistan

D.F. Stepanov (1968, 1969, 1970, 1974) inspected the synanthropic animals of the country for schistosomiasis. Schistosomiasis was quite common for the sheep and cattle of the Dashoguz oasis. The average rate of infection was 40.3% in the cattle and 12.6% in the sheep. Talking about the seasonal variation in the rate of infection with the disease in the sheep and cattle, the author noted that in some seasons the infection rate grew, while in others it became smaller.

Generally, schistosomiasis can be detected in animals in any season, the disease reaching its maximum in autumn and winter and decreasing slightly in spring and summer [33].

Thus, the information provided above on the distribution of schistosomiasis among animals in Central Asia allows us to identify the following zones:

1. Zones with a high level of the extensiveness of schistosomiasis in synanthropic and wild animals—Uzbekistan.

2. Zones with a high infection rate in synanthropic animals—Turkmenistan and Kazakhstan.

3. Zones with relatively weak extensiveness of infection in synanthropic animals—Kyrgyzstan.

In order to carry out a comparative analysis of the epizootology of schistosomiasis in animals, we provide materials for other regions.

5. The Republic of Kazakhstan

In 1909, K.I. Skrjabin detected a parasite in the bifurcations of the portal vein, which, after closer examination, proved to be a new representative of blood flakes. In 1913, the scientist described it and named it *Schistosomum turkestanicum* Skrjabin, 1913.

N.P. Popov (1926) detected five specimens of this trematode in the blood vessels of a cat (*Felis catus* dom.) on the Muynak Island of the Aral Sea. The discovered trematodes were males having no females in their gynecophoral canal.

This trematode was reported to be found in cattle and camels in the territory of Kazakhstan [3, 52–55].

Studying helminthes and helminthiases in the animals of Kazakhstan, S.N. Boyev (1939, 1944) noted that the parasite causing schistosomiasis was a common one and, no doubt, played an important part in animal pathology.

L.I. Lavrov (1963, 1964, 1966) carried out comprehensive research into schistosomiasis, noting that *Sch. turkestanicum* was distributed only within the southern portion of the northern hemisphere (not reaching farther than the 50th parallel) and that schistosoma concentrated in certain areas within their habitat. This parasite was recorded mainly in the animals living close to shores and in slow waters, that is, within the habitats of freshwater molluscs—their intermediate hosts. The trematodes under study are common for the flood plain of the lower course of the Syrdarya River, where the infection rate in cattle equals 26% (reaching 39% in some areas). The infection rate in the middle course of the Syrdarya and its tributary Arys is much lower—2.1%. *Schistosoma* of cattle can be found in any season. The winter infection rate is 28.3% in young animals and 25.3% in mature ones. The number of trematode specimens found in the young animals ranged from 45 to 660 and in the adult ones—from 25 to 237.

Schistosoma can parasitise calves and animals over 10 years of age. The seasonal variation of the infection rate also remains almost the same; however, in young animals, it grows slightly from spring towards winter, while mature animals demonstrate the lowering of the rate [56].

The literary data on schistosomiasis in Kazakhstan show that the regions in the middle course of the Syrdarya are problematic in this respect, with synanthropic animals demonstrating the highest infection rate.

6. The Republic of Azerbaijan

B. Kasimov (1942), S.M. Tuayev (1946) and N.M. Kolesnikov (1953) all together implemented research into the schistosomiasis of animals. According to S.M. Tuayev (1946), trematode *Sch. turkestanicum* causing schistosomiasis was found in the zebu of Lenkoran, Astoran and Massali Districts of Azerbaijan. The author examined 23 zebu (10 of which were from Iran) and 2 buffaloes. Neither of the dissected buffaloes demonstrated traces of *Schistosoma*. As for the zebu, 7 of the inspected animals proved infected. The number of trematode specimens found in the Iranian zebu ranged from 1 to 14, while that in the Azerbaijani ones ranged from 2 to 7838. The parasites were discovered in the mesentery vessels, under the mucous membrane of the small and large intestines, the liver, lungs and spleen.

7. The Russian Federation: the Far East

This zone includes Primorsky and Khabarovsk Krais (borders), Amur, Magadan and Sakhalin Provinces and the Sakha (Yakutia) Republic.

For the first time, the animals of the Far East were inspected for schistosomiasis in 1923, during the 60th USSR Helminthological Expedition headed by Academician K.I. Skrjabin. One of the trematodes causing schistosomiasis, *Sch. bomfordi* (Skrjabin, 1951), was found in sheep.

P.G. Oshmarin (1963) also recorded schistosomiasis (*Sch. turkestanicum*) in the sheep and cattle of the Far East. The average infection rate was 6.4% in sheep and 20.5% in cattle. Some animals were recorded to have died of schistosomiasis. K.G. Abramov (1963) reported about *Schistosoma* in the blood of the elks of the Amur River area.

Ya.N. Zakhryalov (1964–1975) carried out comprehensive research into schistosomiasis of the animals of the Far East. In 1975, the researcher established that the average infection rate in Primorsky was 22.9% in cattle and 6.5% in sheep. *Schistosoma* had spread over a large area, which, in the author's opinion, is conditioned by the broad network of water bodies covering the territory of the region.

Ya.N. Zakhryalov (1964, 1972, 1975) studied the seasonal variations of the rate of infection with schistosomiasis in the cattle of the upper Amur River area and Primorsky. The author noted that, unlike in Uzbekistan, Kazakhstan and Iran, the rate of infection with schistosomiasis and the number of *Schistosoma* specimens in the cattle of the Far East varies greatly depending on the age, growing strongly between the age of 5 months and 3 years (0.5–2.6% in calves, 9.8–16.2% in youngsters over 1 year and 30.5–34.4% in adults). The average infection rate in mature animals between 3 and 7 years old was equal to 28.0%, between 7 and 10–28.5%, and between 11 and 18–27.3%.

Schistosoma's definitive hosts in this region, unlike in other territories, are synanthropic animals and some of the wild ones, such as the elk, reindeer and Siberian roe deer, which makes the epizootic situation connected with schistosomiasis quite unique in the Far East.

The average rate of infection with schistosomiasis in the domestic animals of the CIS (Commonwealth of Independent States) countries is higher than that in the wild animals.

Here we should note that currently, domestic animals play a much greater role in the transmission and circulation of schistosomiasis than wild animals do. However, it is obvious that in the recent past wild animals played an important part in the transmission of schistosomiasis to synanthropic ones.

Having an idea about the general picture of *Sch. turkestanicum*'s distribution in the countries of the former USSR, we thought it expedient to analyse this problem in other countries across Asia and Europe.

Ye.Ye. Shumakovich (1936) recorded *Sch. turkestanicum* in the cattle and dzo of **Mongolia**. '...the parasite's location in the blood vessels of the liver makes us think that this guest cannot be harmless to its host, the more so as its close relations parasitising humans cause a serious disease – schistosomiasis. The history and epizootology of the disease in cattle remain completely unstudied, and neither preventive measure no cure has been developed'. This *Schistosoma* is also reported to be found in the domestic animals of Mongolia [57, 58].

M.F. Hsü (1938) noted a widespread schistosomiasis in sheep and goats in Xinjiang, Gansu, Ningxia, Suiyuan and Hubei provinces of the **People's Republic of China**. The author also reported about cercarioses of humans, which were caused by *Sch. turkestanicum* cercariae in the Chinese wetlands, where schistosomiasis is quite common. Kuo (Skrjabin, 1951) recorded schistosomiasis in cattle in one of the Chinese provinces, where the infection rate reached 40.0%. Lien Chien-an et al. (1975) established that in 1965 35% of the inspected cattle were recorded to be infected with blood flukes, with four animal specimens being parasitised by *Sch. turkestanicum*. The authors established that *Radix ovata*, *R. lagotis* and *Galba laticallosiformis* are the trematode's intermediate hosts.

C.T. Tang et al. (1983, 1990, 1990a,b) carried out comprehensive research into *Sch. turkestanicum* parasitising sheep and goats. The researcher determined the infection rate, which did not exceed 6.8% and its seasonal variations. From July to September cercariae of *Sch. turkestanicum* were found in infected molluscs. The work provides data on the parasites' superficial structure, which were obtained using scanning electron microscopy. In particular, the author indicated the structural changes in this trematode occurring at different ages. He noted that 93.8–99.2% of the parasites from the dissected sheep were found in mesenteric veins.

MacHattie (1936) studied schistosomiasis in animals in different regions of **Iraq**. The author reported that the infection rate in the sheep, goats and cattle of the wetlands along the banks of the Tigris reached 80%, while that in the horses, donkeys, mules and camels is 15.0%.

Schistosomiasis is also quite common in **Iran**, where it was recorded both in wild and in synanthropic animals (cattle, sheep, goats, buffaloes, camels and wild boars) [23, 59] established that the infection rate was 30% in cattle, 16% in sheep, 7% in goats and 2% in buffaloes.

Dut and Srivastava (1952, 1955, 1961); Kumar (1973); Chauhan et al. (1973); Singh, Ahluwalia (1977); Srivastava, Kumar (1990); Agrawal et al. (1991); Mukherjee (2007) studied *Sch. turkestanicum* and *Sch. dattai* parasitising cattle, buffaloes, sheep, goats, horses, donkeys, mules and camels in **India**.

M. Abdussalam and M. Sarwar (1953) recorded *Sch. turkestanicum* in the sheep and goats of **Pakistan**. S. Yasin (1959) reported that parasitic diseases caused theheaviest material loss to Pakistan's cattle breeding. He referred *Sch. turkestanicum* causing schistosomiasis to pathogenic trematodes.

Witenberg, Lengy (1966) report about *Sch. turkestanicum* found in rats and sheep in **Turkey**.

There was a report from G. Marotel (1908) about schistosomiasis in the cattle of **France**.

And, finally, G. Majoros et al. (2010) report on finding *Sch. turkestanicum* in a European red deer in **Hungary**.

The cercariae of *Sch. turkestanicum* are known to cause such diseases as dermatitis and cercarioses in nonspecific hosts [3, 11, 12, 29, 30, 42, 49, 60–65].

Therefore, *Sch. turkestanicum* in synanthropic and natural centres of infection should be regarded as a problem important from the epizootological and epidemiological aspects [7, 42].

At the end of the survey of *Sch. turkestanicum* in various domestic and wild animals in different countries around the world, we should refer to the report of doctor P. Vittoz (1959). The author considers schistosomiasis caused by this trematode the principal disease of zebu and buffaloes in a number of Asian countries (India, Sri Lanka, Pakistan, Burma, Thailand, Laos, Cambodia, Vietnam and Indonesia). These materials testify to the damage the disease causes to the economies of these countries. It is obvious that this fact has resulted in the growing number of publications on this infection in animals in some Asian countries.

A number of researchers [20, 66–68] reported about the use of histological and histochemical methods in the examination of *Sch. turkestanicum.*

L.I. Lavrov (1974) used the histochemical method to inspect the tissues of this *Schistosoma* for copper, iron, protein and tryptophan. The author suggested that the characteristics of the trematode, thus, obtained should be used for the development of effective remedies for this type of helminthiasis.

Researchers reported pathological changes in the cuticle and intestine of *Sch. turkestanicum* on the 3rd, 5th, 6th and 15th days after they had been given therapeutic doses of chloxylum (150 mg/kg, twice with an interval of 24 hours) and thiabendazole (600 mg/kg) to rabbits infected artificially with the experimental purpose [67]. The authors noted that, affected by chloxylum, the cuticle swells, becomes vaculated in places and disintegrates; the intestine also swells, the syncytium cytoplasm becomes friable and the fibrous basal membrane roughens. Thiabendazole causes the complete disappearance of cuticular thorns from the surface of the parasite's body. The same authors (1978) gave the original materials on the micromorphology of the covering cuticle, oesophagus, intestine, vitelline and seminal glands, ovary and eggs, as well on the distribution of nucleic acids in the parasite's different organs. The difference lies in the structure of the digestive tract of males and females, which depends on the way they feed. *Sch. turkestanicum* females are characterised by intestinal digestion with intercellular elements, while males feed somatically in most cases.

The work provided data on the ultrastructure of the cuticle and entodermal canal of *Sch. turkestanicum*. According to the authors, the cuticle is similar in structure to the canal. It is penetrated by a number of narrow canals, which are divided into three types, according to structure and size—they are hollow but are filled with electron-dense granules, similar to the granules of the erythrocyte cytoplasm of the definitive host. The entodermal canal is covered with a layer of gland cells similar to syncytia. The cytoplasmic membrane of the gland cell facing the lumen of the canal forms, together with numerous folds, villous projections with villi directed to the intestine's cavity, which, contracting, pull particles of food into the cytoplasm, forming food vacuoles in it. The researchers consider that the cuticle of the male *Schistosoma* is connected with the metabolic function.

Z. Zdarska et al. (1986) studied the histochemistry of *Sch. turkestanicum* cercariae. Using histochemical methods, they identified four types of gland cells in this trematode: the outlet, head, preacetabular and postacetabular glands. The head gland secretion contains proteins with cystine and cysteine, and phospholipids, showing the activity of acid phosphatase. The outlet gland secretion contains proteins with cystine and cysteine, the postacetabular gland secretion—proteins with cystine, cysteine and tyrosine, and central and acid flour substances.

L.I. Lavrov and E.D. Daugaliyeva (1988) described pathologic histological changes in the organs of rabbits infected with various quantities of *Sch. turkestanicum*. The pathologic histological changes depended upon the number of parasite specimens. The heaviest abnormalities were recorded in the liver and small intestine. M. Isayev (1995) noted similar abnormalities in his works.

According to R. Khegner (1937), parasitology regards the parasite and host as a uniform biological system, which resulted from the evolutionary adaptation of the parasite to its host and which is characterised by special relations, which are called the 'host-parasite relationships'. The host's organism is the parasite's habitat. That is why the parasite has adapted to the host's metabolism in the course of its evolution. The 'parasite-host' system is characterised by close relations, and although the organism's function more or less separately, the metabolism of one of them depends on the other or is regulated by it.

The parasite's and host's metabolism, and particularly the lipidic one, is of certain interest and, therefore, the biochemical mechanisms regulating the stability of the 'parasite-host' system should be studied closer.

It is interesting that helminths' lipids join with proteins to protect the latter from being digested by enzymes and endow them with a number of toxic properties [69]. Therefore, to study this group is important not only from the scientific aspect but also from the practical one.

In recent years active investigation has been made into the phospholipids of parasitic worms. This is connected with the insufficiency of information on the composition and biosynthesis of phospholipids in helminthes, in particular, in trematodes [70–73]. Most of the phospholipids are phosphatidylcholine and phosphatidylethanolamine. The total amounts of these two fractions may be between 60% and 85% of the total phospholipids in some helminths, where the portion of phosphatidylcholine is usually 1.5–3.0 as large as that of phosphatidylethanolamine. Other phospholipid fractions are present in small quantities.

Let us enlarge slightly upon the phospholipid and fatty-acid compositions in trematodes from the family Schistosomatidae.

In adult trematodes *S. mansoni* phospholipids comprise 20-30 % of the total amount of lipids (Smith, Brooks, 1969). Most of the phospholipids are phosphatidylcholine and phosphatidylethanolamine. These fractions comprise 60–85% of the total amount of phospholipids.

F. Meyer et al. (1970) maintained that they did not discover phosphatidyl serine, sphingomyelin and lysolecitin in trematode *S. mansoni*.

It should be noted that, although flatworms contain large amounts of unsaturated fatty acids and sterols, they are not capable of synthesising these compounds (Meyer et al., 1966; Smith, Brooks, 1969). This information can be treated differently. It may be a characteristic metabolic feature for all flatworms. It may be a manifestation of the worms' adaptation to the parasitic lifestyle. And, finally, it may result from the anaerobic conditions intestinal parasites live in. We know that animals need oxygen for the biosynthesis of sterols and unsaturated fatty acids.

To come to one definite conclusion F. Meyer et al. (1970) carried out an experiment on a parasite living in an oxygen environment (*S. mansoni*) and a non-parasitic flatworm (turbellarian worm *Dudesia dorotocephala*), to study the lipid biosynthesis. The qualitative compositions proved to be almost the same in both worms, although the quantities of the compounds were a little different. Most of the lipids in both worms consist of cholesterol, triglycerides and phospholipids. The principal fatty acids are unsaturated, monoene and polyene acids containing 16–22 carbon atoms.

The researchers established that both flatworms lost the ability to synthesise *de novo* sterols and long-chain fatty acids. However, the worms can synthesise lipids with the help of fatty acids and sterols that they take with food.

The works of W. Bruce and B. Ronald (1984) provide data on the phospholipid composition in the cercariae and adults of *S. mansoni*. The total amount of phospholipids (in one mg of proteins) was considerably larger in adults. Phosphatidylcholine was the predominant phospholipid in adults, while phosphatidylethanolamine was the principal phospholipid in cercariae. The portions of almost all phospholipids, except for phosphatidylglycerol and phosphatidyl inositol, were larger in the adults than in the cercariae.

Naiki Masaharu et al. (1985) provide data on the lipid composition of mature *S. mansoni*, which were obtained from infected people and mice parasitised with cercariae. The phospholipid composition and ratio were the same in both cases. Large amounts of phosphatidylcholine-dyacilglycerin and small quantities of phosphatidyl-ethanol-amindiadyglicerin were recorded in the parasites.

According to A. David et al. (1987), the phospholipid composition in the adults and cercariae of *S. mansoni* and their isolated outer membranes is similar to the phospholipid composition of the membranes of erythrocytes. The predominating fatty acids in the phosphatidylcholine of *S. mansoni* are palmitic and oleic acids, while eicosenoic acid is the main acid in phosphatidylethanolamine and phosphatidyl serine. Large amounts of eicosenoic acid together with hepatopancreas phospholipid were found in uninfected snails *Biomphalaria glabrata*, the intermediate host of *S. mansoni*, while no eicosenoic acid was found in the erythrocytes of uninfected hamsters. *S. mansoni* is supposed to be able to synthesise eicosenoic acid out of oleic acid.

S.T. Furlong and J.P. Caulfield (1989) obtained mechanically schistosomula from *S. mansoni* cercariae and then bred them *in vitro*. To determine the syntheses of different lipids and to study them in a culture medium the researchers added marked predecessors of lipids, such as choline, ethanolamine, palmitate and oleate, into this medium and then checked the contents of the marked substances in different lipids. The authors noted the ability of schistosomula to synthesise monopalmitoyl-phosphatidylcholine, which plays an important part in the protection of schistosomula from their host's immunity and emit it actively into the environment.

In the end of this survey, we should note that in literary sources we have not found any information on the phospholipid and fatty acid composition of trematode *Sch. turkestanicum*.

The problem of the impact of trematode parthenitae on their intermediate hosts, freshwater molluscs, has been discussed sufficiently in literary sources [74–82].

It should be noted that in most cases trematode larvae inhabit the molluscs' digestive gland (liver)—an organ that participates actively in the synthesis, modification and excretion of various lipids. Molluscs infected with treamatode parthenitae suffer various metabolic disturbances. Thus, phospholipid metabolism results in a change in the total amount of phospholipids and their fractions. Literary data on this issue is scarce and disputable.

According to T. Reader (1976), the parasitised digestive gland of intermediate hosts contains larger portions of neutral fats and fatty acids, which result from the disintegration of the molluscs' fats affected by the parasites' lipase. The number of phospholipids grows considerably in the hepatopancreas of molluscs *Littorina saxatilis* parasitised with parthenitae [83]. Cheng also noted that fact earlier; he also mentioned the decrease in the portion of fats in Leydig's cells in infected oysters.

In his works, O.V. Guminsky (1984) compares data on the content of total lipids, triglycerides and cholesterol in the hemolymph of *Viviparus viviparus* and *Lymnaea stagnalis* infected and uninfected with trematode parthenitae. He established that the content of lipids in the hemolymph of Viviparidae infected with parthenitae and metacercariae of *Echinoparyphium petrowi* and pond snails with parthenitae and metacercariae of *E. aconiatum* does not change. This testifies to a high resistance of molluscs' lipid metabolism to trematodes.

B.I. James (1965) considers that the phospholipid deficit in molluscs' organs infected with parthenitae is conditioned by their host's use of them as a source of energy, as parthenitae and trematode larvae utilise most of their host's glycogen, which serves as their reserve energy source.

Th. Cheng, Th. James H. (1960), Patnaik, Ray (1960), Porter et al. (1967), A.P. Stadnichenko (1968, 1972), I.P. Yavorsky (1989) provide information on the decrease of phospholipid contents in the hepatopancreas and gonads of molluscs infected with trematode parthenitae.

In literary sources, we did not find information on the composition of phospholipid in the tissues of either uninfected molluscs *L. auricularia* or molluscs parasitised with *Sch. turkestanicum* parthenitae.

Using the above-given data on phospholipids' role in the membrane, and compensatory and adaptive processes in organisms in extreme conditions we studied the phospholipid and fatty acid composition of mature trematode *Sch. turkestanicum*, the content of phospholipid fractions and fatty acids in the liver of molluscs *L. auricularia* and the parasite's influence on the content of the mentioned components in cattle's liver. In addition, we have studied the proteins of blood serum and the physical and chemical changes in the blood of animals infected experimentally.

To summarise, specialists from a number of scientific fields, such as zoology, parasitology and related, have become increasingly more interested in the study of trematodes *Sch. turkestanicum* in recent years. We attempted to generalise the sporadic data published in various sources [7]. We took into account the inaccessibility of the Russian version of the monograph for international researchers and thought that it is also reasonable to publish an abridged variant of the book in English.

Author details

Djalaliddin A. Azimov, Firuza D. Akramova and Ulugbek A. Shakarbaev
Institute of Zoology of the Academy of Sciences of the Republic of Uzbekistan, Tashkent, Uzbekistan

*Address all correspondence to: safarov-alisher@mail.ru

References

[1] Dutt SC, Srivastava HD. A revision of the genus *Ornithobilharzia* Odner 1912 (Trematoda: Schistosomatidae). Proceedings of the Indian Science Congress. 1955;**42**:61-73

[2] Price EW. A synopsis of the Trematode family Schistosomidae with descriptions of new Genera and Species. Proceedings of the United States National Museum. 1929;**75**(Art.18):1-39

[3] Skrjabin KI. Trematodes of Animals and Human. The Principles of Trematodology. Vol. 5. Moscow: Nauka; 1951. p. 622

[4] Dutt SC, Srivastava HD. Studies on the life history of *Orientobilharzia turkestanica* (Skrjabin, 1913) Dutt and Srivastava, 1955. Current Science. 1964;**22**(24):752-753

[5] Chauhan AS, Srivastava CB, Chauhan BS. Studies on the trematode fauna of India. Part 6. Digenea: Schistosomatidae. A monographie aid to the identification of Indian schistosomes. Journal of the Zoological Society of India. 1973;**25**(12):83-127

[6] Azimov DA. The Schistosomes of Animals and Humans. Tashkent: Fan; 1975. 152 p

[7] Azimov DA, Akramova FD, Shakarbaev UA, Shakarboyev EB. Orientobildgarsii - mammalian trematodes. Tashkent: Fan; 2014. 224 p

[8] Snyder SD, Loker ES. Evolutionary relationships among the Schistosomatidae (Platyhelminthes: Digenea) and an Asian origin for Schistosoma. Parasitology. 2000;**86**:283-288

[9] Lockyer AE, Olson PD, Littlewood DTJ. Utility of complete large and small subunit rRNA genes in resolving the phylogeny of the Platyhelminthes: Implications and review of the cercomer theory. Biologikal Journal of the Linnean Society. 2003;**78**:155-173

[10] Li L, Yu LY, Zhu XQ, Wang CR, Zhai YQ, Zhao JP. Orientobilharzia turkestanicum is grouped within African schistosomes based on phylogenetic analyses using sequences of mitochondrial genes. Parasitology Research. 2008;**102**:939-943

[11] Wang CR, Li L, Ni HB, Zhai YQ, Chen AH, Cheh J, et al. *Orientobilharzia turkestanica* is a member of *Schistosoma* genus based on phylogenetic analysis using ribosomal DNA sequences. Experimental Parasitology. 2009;**121**:193-197

[12] Majoros G, Dan A, Erdelyi K. A natural focus of the blood fluke *Orientobilharzia turkestanica* (Skrjabin, 1913) (Trematoda: Schistosomatidae) in red deer (*Cervus elaphus*) in Hungery. Veterinary Parasitology. 2010;**170**(3-4): 218-223

[13] Witenberg GC, Lengy J. A case of natural infection of field rats with *Ornithobilharzia turkestanica*. Refuah Veterinarith. 1966;**23**(1):64-67

[14] Zakhryalov YN. *Orientobilharzia turkestanica* (Skrjabin, 1913) Dutt and Srivastava, 1955 in the Far East: The abstract of a doctoral thesis. Alma-Ata: Institute of Zoology; 1975. p. 43

[15] Skrjabin KI. *Schistosomum turkestanicum* n. sp., ein newer Parasit des Rindes aus Russischen-Turkestan.

Zeitschr. fur Infectionskrankheiten, parasitare Krankheiten und Hygiene der Haustiere. 1913;**13**(7):458-468

[16] MacHattie C. A preliminary note on the life history of *Schistosoma turkestanicum* Skrjabin, 1913. Transactions of the Royal Society of Tropical Medicine & Hygiene. 1936;**30**:115-124

[17] Abdussalam M, Sarwar MM. Schistosomiasis in Pakistan. In: XVth International Veterinary Congress. Peshawar: 1953. Part I. pp. 18-23

[18] Lavrov LI. The rate of infection with *Ornithobilharzia* in the cattle of South Kazakhstan. Parasites of the Agricultural Animals of Kazakhstan: Alma-Ata. 1964;**3**:108-113

[19] Arfaa F, Sabaghian H, Ale - Bawood H. Studies on *Orientobilharzia turkestanica* (Skrjabin, 1913) Price, 1929 in Iran. Annales de Parasitologie Humaine et Comparee. 1965;**40**:45-50

[20] Lavrov LI, Daugaliyeva EK. The Impact of Orientobilharziasis Intensity on the Pathologic Process. Moscow: The All-USSR Institute of Helminthology; 1988. pp. 79-88

[21] Kumar V. Studies on snail hosts of *Orientobilharzia turkestanicum* (Skrjabin, 1913) Dutt et Srivastava, 1955 (Schistosomatidae: Trematoda) in India. Annales de la Société Belge de Médecine Tropicale. 1973;**53**(1):17-23

[22] Massoud J. Studies on the schistosomes of domestic animals in Iran. I. Observations on *Orientobilharzia turkestanica* (Skrjabin, 1913) in Khuzestan. Journal of Helminthology. 1973;**67**(2):165-180

[23] Massoud J. The effect of variations in miracidial exposure dose on laboratory infections of *Ornithobilharzia turkestanica* in *Lymnaea gedrosiana*. Journal of Helminthology. 1974;**48**(2):139-144

[24] Zakhryalov YN. The intermediate host of *Ornithobilharzia turkestanica* (Skrjabin, 1913) in the Far East. In: The Materials of a Scientific Conference. Part. 1. Moscow: Nauka; 1965. pp. 90-95

[25] Zakhryalov YN. The Forms of Association of *Ornithobilharzia Turkestanica* with Specific Definitive Hosts. Blagoveshchensk: Nauka; 1974. pp. 61-71

[26] Azimov DA. To the epizotology of orientobilharziasis in the ruminants of Uzbekistan. In: The Materials of a Scientific Conference. Part. 1. Moscow: Nauka; 1966. pp. 3-7

[27] Azimov D.A. On the relation of trematode *Ornithobilharzia turkestanica* (Skrjabin, 1913) to specific hosts. The Materials of a Scientific Conference. Moscow, 1971. pp. 6-10

[28] Azimov DA. On the habitats of trematodes from the genus *Orientobilharzia*. The Uzbek Biological Magazine. Tashkent: Fan; 1978;(3):44-46

[29] Sahba Gholam HA, Malek EA. Dermatitis caused by cercariae of *Orientobilharzia turkestanica* in the Caspian Sea area of Iran. American Journal of Tropical Medicine and Hygiene. 1979;**28**(5):912-912

[30] Amid A, Gohar S, Rosnami M. Dermination of definitive and intermediate hosts of cercarial dermatitis-producing agents in northern Iran. Archives of Iranian Medicine. 2006;**9**(1):11-15

[31] Azimov DA. Freshwater mollusc *Radix auricularia* as the intermediate host of *Orientobilharzia turkestanica*

in Uzbekistan. The Uzbek Biological Magazine. 1968;(4):42-44

[32] Panin VY, Lavrov LI, Uvaliyeva KK. The study of the life cycle of *Orientobilharzia turkestanica* (Skrjabin, 1913). In: The Materials of the Conference Dedicated to the Memory of N. V. Badanin. Tashkent: Fan; 1968. pp. 246-247

[33] Stepanov DF. Ornitobilharziosis of animals in Turkmen SSR and the experimental therapy of this helminthiasis: The abstract of a PhD thesis in the veterinary science. M; 1969. 18 p

[34] Zakhryalov YN. The ways of the infction of the definitive host with *Ornithobilharzia turkestanica*. Part 1. Moscow: Nauka; 1968. pp. 118-122

[35] Zakhryalov YN. On the Biology of *Orientobilharzia Turkestanica* (Skrjabin, 1913) in the Far East. Natural Diseases and the Questions of Parasitology in the Republics of Central Asia and Kazakhstan. Almaty: Donish; 1969. pp. 155-158

[36] Zakhryalov YN. To the question of the posthumous diagnostics of orientobilharziasis caused by *Ornithobilharzia turkestanica*. In: The Materials of the 18th Scientific Conference. Blagoveshchensk: Nauka; 1970. pp. 82-84

[37] Azimov DA, Dadayev S. The daily biological rhythms of cercariae's emission. Reports by the Academy of Sciences. Tashkent: Fan; 1977;(5):67-69

[38] Azimov DA. The specificities of the life cycle of *Ornithobilharzia turkestanica* (Skrjabin, 1913) in Uzbekistan. In: The Materials of a Scientific Conference. Moscow: Nauka; 1968. pp. 7-14

[39] Uvaliyeva KK, Lavrov LI. The epizootological role of pond snails in different water bodies of the south and southeast of Kazakhstan in the distribution of orientobilharziosis. In: The Materials of the 2nd Transcaucasian Conference for Parasitology. Yerevan: The Academy of Sciences of Armenia; 1981. pp. 233-234

[40] Azimov DA, Nurmukhamedov KN. Orientobilharziasis in ruminants. Journal Agriculture of Uzbekistan. Tashkent: Mekhnat. 1967;(7):56-58

[41] Azimov DA, Nurmukhamedov KN. New data on the biology of trematode *Orientobilharzia turkestanica* (Schistosomatidae). The Zoological Magazine. 1968;(10):1471-1478

[42] Azimov DA, Arifjanov ZK. Research into the blood serum proteins of sheep infected experimentally with orientobilharziasis. In: The Works of All-Russian Skrjabin Scientific Research Institute of Helmonthology. Moscow; 1969. pp. 25-32

[43] Azimov DA, Sultanov MA, Dadayev S. On helminths of the domestic animals of Jizzakh Province. The Uzbek Biological Magazine. Tashkent: Fan; 1979;(6):54-57

[44] Arkhipov IA. Mixed infection in the cattle of Karakalpakistan. The Materials of the 10th Conference of the Ukrainian Parasitologists' Society. 1988;**4**(3):9-10

[45] Shakiyev YS. The prevention of orientobilharziasis of animals in the Karakalpaki ASSR. helminthology today: Problems and prospects. In: The Thesis of the Report of a Scientific Conference. Part 2. M; 1989. p. 168

[46] Salimov BS, Shamsiyev BM, Mukumov K. Mixed diseases of cattle caused by trematodes and the questions of their prevention in the Aral Sea area. In: The Collection of Scientific Treatises "the Prevention and Treatment of

Infectious Diseases in Hot Climates". Tashkent: Fan; 1990. pp. 45-49

[47] Isayev M. The pathomorphological changes in cattle infected with orientobilharziasis: The abstract of a doctoral thesis. Samarkand: 1995. p. 19

[48] Shakarboyev EB. The ecological and functional interrelations of *Orientobilharzia turkestanica* (Skrjabin, 1913) – *Bos taurus* Linnaeus, 1758 in the parasite-host system: A PhD thesis in biology. Tashkent: 1996. p. 134

[49] Shakarboyev EB. Trematodes of the vertebrates of Uzbekistan (the species composition, circulation ways, ecology ad biology): A doctoral thesis in biology. Tashkent: 2009. p. 243

[50] Azimov DA. *Ornithobilharzia Turkestanica* (Skrjabin, 1913) in Sheep and Cattle. A Treatise Issued by Uzbek Scientific and Research Institute. Tashkent: Fan; 1965;**17**:9-10

[51] Azimov DA. To the study of orientobilharziasis in the sheep, goats and cattle of Uzbekistan. The materials of a scientific conference. Всесоюзного общество гельминтов АН СССР. Moscow: Nauka; 1965. Part. 2. P. 8-9

[52] Wolf ZV. On the characteristics of the helminthic fauna in the cattle of Kazakhstan. 1936(1):73-76

[53] Panova LG. Helminthology in Kazakhstan. A Collection of Works in Helminthology. Moscow: Science; 1927. pp. 121-137

[54] Panova LG. To the Question of Distribution of Cattle's Orientobilharziasis in Kazakhstan. Kazakh Scientific Research Institute of Veterinary Science. 1940;**3**:428-430

[55] Pryadko EI. The Rate of Infection with Helminths in the Cattle of Southeast Kazakhstan. The Parasites of the Agricultural Animals of Kazakhstan. Alma-Ata: Ilim. 1962;(1):134-154

[56] Lavrov LI, Fedoseyenko VM. The Ultrastructure of the Cuticle and Intestinal Tube of *Orientobilharzia Turkestanica* (Skrjabin, 1913). The Life Cycles, Ecology and Morphology of Helminthes in the Animals of Kazakhstan. Alma-Ata: Science; 1978. pp. 88-94

[57] Ivashkin VM. Helminths of the Agricultural Animals of Mongolia. Moscow: Science; 1955. pp. 14-16

[58] Yamagiva S. A study of lesions caused by the invasion of *Schistosomum turkestanicum* Skrjabin, 1913 in cattle. Journal of The Japanese Society of Veterinary Science. 1931;**10**(2):128-132

[59] Massoud J, Nelson GS. The study of the heteroimmunity of beings infected with schistosomiasis. The Bulletin of WHO. Geneva. 1973;**47**(5):572-580

[60] Hsü HF. *Schistosoma turkestanicum* in North China. Chinese Medical Journal. 1938;**54**:568-578

[61] Plotnikov NN. A Disease Caused by Flukes (Trematodes). Contagious Diseases of Human. Moscow: Medicina; 1955. pp. 551-556

[62] Zakhryalov YN. On the Methods of Testing Anti-Orientobilharziasis Medicines on Rabbits. The Questions of Scientific Research Methods in the Agriculture of Siberia and the Far East. Novosibirsk: Nauka; 1972. pp. 150-152

[63] Chien-An L, Kung-Mao P, Lung S, Chao-Ming L, Min-Sen C, Chung L. A survey of the aetiological agent of rice-field dermatitis in Chegnan peoples commune, Hailung Hsien, Kirin Province,

with a preliminary observation of the life history of *Orientobilharzia turkestanica* var. tuberculata. Dunu syuabao. Acta Zoologica Sinica. 1975;**21**(2):183-189

[64] Azimov DA. Tremadodes—Parasites of Animals and Human. Tashkent: Mehnat; 1986. 128 p

[65] Azimov DA, Shakarboyev EB, Isakova DT, Akramova FD. Parazitologiya terminlarni izokhli lugati. Tashkent: Fan; 2007. p. 210

[66] Lavrov LI. The Copper, Iron, Proteins and Tryptophan Contents in the Tissues of Ornithobilharzia. The Materials for the Republican Seminar-Conference for the Control of Parasitic and Non-Contagious Diseases Agricultural Animals. Alma-Ata: Nauka; 1974. pp. 184-187

[67] Lavrov LI, Koshkina NG. The Micromorphological Study of *Ornithobilharzia Turkestanica* before and after Treatment with Anti-Helminthic Agents. The Problems of the Experimental Morphological Physiology and Genetics. Kemerovo: Nauka; 1976. pp. 157-160

[68] Lavrov LI, Koshkina NG. The Histological Inspection of *Ornithobilharzia Turkestanica*. The Life Cycles, Ecology and Morphology of Helminthes in the Animals of Kazakhstan. Alma-Ata: Nauka; 1978. pp. 78-87

[69] Yarygina GV. The Lipids of Trematode Paramphistomum cervi. The Research into the Fauna, Taxonomy and Biochemistry of the Helminths of the Far East. Vladivostok: Nauka; 1972. pp. 199-203

[70] Smith TM, Brooks TJ. Lipid fractions in adult Schistosoma mansoni. Parasitology. 1969;**59**(2):293-298

[71] Meyer F, Meyer H, Bueding I. Lipid metabolism in the parasitic and free—Living flatworms *Schistosoma mansoni* and *Dugesia dorotocephala*. Biochimica et Biophysica Acta. 1970;**210**(2):257-260

[72] Bruce W, Ronald B. Phospholipids of cercariae and adult *Schistosoma mansoni*. The Journal of Parasitology. 1984;**70**(3):447-448

[73] David A, Gilberto P, Evans W, Howard. The phospholipid and fatty acid composition of *Schistosoma mansoni* and of its purified tedumental membranes. Molecular and Biochemical Parasitology. 1987;**22**(2):123-128

[74] Ginetsinskaya TA. Trematodes, their Life Cycles, Biology and Evolution. L: Nauka; 1968. 411 p

[75] Christie JD, Foster WB, Stauber LA. The effect of parasitism and starvation on carbohydrate reserves of *Biomphalaria glabrata*. Journal of Invertebrate Pathology. 1974;**22**(1):55-62

[76] Bear SA. The "parasite-host" relations in the "mollusc-trematodes" system. The Achievements of Contemporary Biology. 1978;**1**(4):86, 143-153

[77] Stadnichenko AP. Phospholipids in the digestive gland of molluscs infected with trematode larvae. Parasitology. 1968;**2**:35-37

[78] Stadnichenko AP. The pathogenic impact of trematode parthenitae on freshwater molluscs. The Hydrobiological Magazine. 1977;**13**(1):117-124

[79] Stadnichenko AP. Interrelations in the "host (freshwater mollusc) – Parasite (trematodes)" system. The Hydrobiological Magazine. 1984;**15**(6):31-36

[80] Guminsky OV. The impact of trematode parthenitae on the lipid

metabolism of freshwater molluscs. Parasitology. 1984;**19**(4):306-309

[81] Yavorsky IP. Relations in the system "*Fasciola hepatica – Lymnaea (Galba) truncatula*". Parasitology. 1989;**23**(4):355-357

[82] Hurd H. Physiological and behavioural interactions between parasites and invertebrate hosts. Advoncesin Parasitology. 1990;**29**(1):148-149

[83] Bear SA. The "parasite-host" relations in the "mollusc-trematodes" system. The Achievements of Contemporary Biology. 1978;**86**(4):143-153

Chapter 3

The Materials and Methods of Study

Djalaliddin A. Azimov, Bakhrom T. Norkobilov, Firuza D. Akramova, Ulugbek A. Shakarbaev and Alisher A. Safarov

Abstract

The chapter presents methodological approaches: natural observations and conducting experimental studies. Traditional methods of research are described: helminthological, parasitological, malacological, and ecological and molecular genetics. Also, much attention is paid to the collection sites of the material, the species composition and the number of animals studied (vertebrates and invertebrates). Preparation of homogenates of trematode *Sch. turkestanicum*, and liver of *Lymnaea auricularia* molluscs was carried out. Methods of thin-layer chromatography, determination of the fatty acid composition of phospholipids, hydrolysis and methylation of phospholipids and their fractions are described. Methods of histological studies of organs of infected animals are highlighted.

Keywords: northwestern, central, eastern, northeastern, southern, Uzbekistan, miracidioscopy, electrophoresis, *Lymnaea auricularia*, *Schistosoma turkestanicum*, homogenate, fractions

1. The Materials and Methods of Study

The material primarily used in this work included, primarily, the results of our own research into the morphology, biology and ecology of trematode *Schistosoma turkestanicum,* which was implemented in 1965–2020. We studied the ecology and fauna of the aquatic and terrestrial conenoses of the Amudarya and Syrdarya river basins and the Aral Sea and made a considerable amount of experimental research. We studied a large number of domestic and wild animals in all the regions of Uzbekistan (**Figure 1**). We collected and examined molluscs from the families Lymnaeidae, Planorbidae and Physidae in different types of water bodies of the above-mentioned rivers. The numbers of studied animals are given in corresponding chapters of the monograph.

In our work, we used the traditional helminthological, malacological and ecological research methods [1–6].

In an effort to study the trematode's life cycle, we used the parasite's eggs from sheep and cattle from the farms of the Republic of Karakalpakstan infected in a natural way.

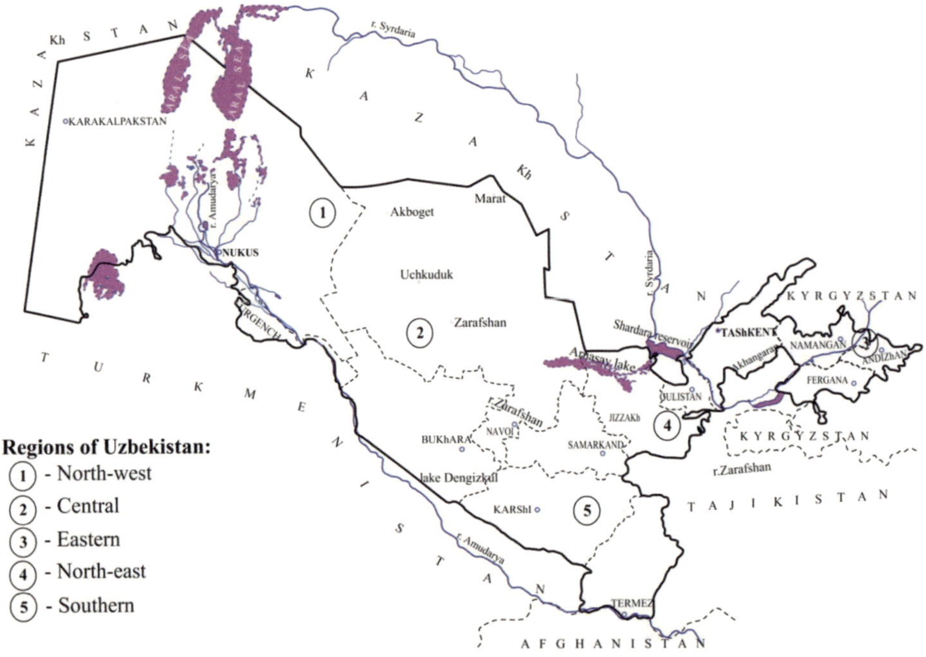

Figure 1.
Map of Uzbekistan: The area where the material was collected.

We used miracidia that emerged from eggs in the laboratory to infect freshwater molluscs. For getting miracidia stage, we developed a special method [7]. The method is based on the presence of positive phototaxis and negative geotaxis in miracidias. The method is simple and suits perfectly collect miracidia (**Figure 2**).

To inspect miracidia, we put 10–15 g of animal faeces into a nylon or gauze bag and placed it into a flask with water heated to a temperature of 30–32°C. The flask had a bent glass pipe 1 cm in diameter soldered to its neck. We covered all the parts of the flask with cardboard.

The glass tube can be illuminated with a lamp. If the bird is infected with Schistosomatidae, in 30–40 minutes we can observe miracidia moving actively in the pipe. Then, using a pipette, we take several drops of water from the upper part of the pipe and place them on a watch glass, cavity slide or Petri dish and observe them using a microscope.

We used molluscs bred in laboratories and collected in bodies of water not visited by animals to infect them experimentally with *Sch. turkestanicum* miracidia. We were infecting the molluscs individually or in groups. When infecting individually, we placed one mollusc and 1 to 3 active miracidia of the same age group into the Petri dishes (we used miracidia that have emerged from eggs 1–2 hours ago). In 24 hours, we transferred the molluscs to small aquaria, 25–30 specimens to each aquarium. When being infected in groups, the molluscs were kept in aquaria, 75–100 specimens in each, where later miracidia were added.

The molluscs were kept in aquaria at different temperatures and fed on grapevine and mulberry leaves.

We used the well-known method [3, 8] to study the morphology and biology of parthenogenetic generations. We studied the morphology and biology of miracidia and cercariae with the use of vital dye. We prepared an anesthetised solution

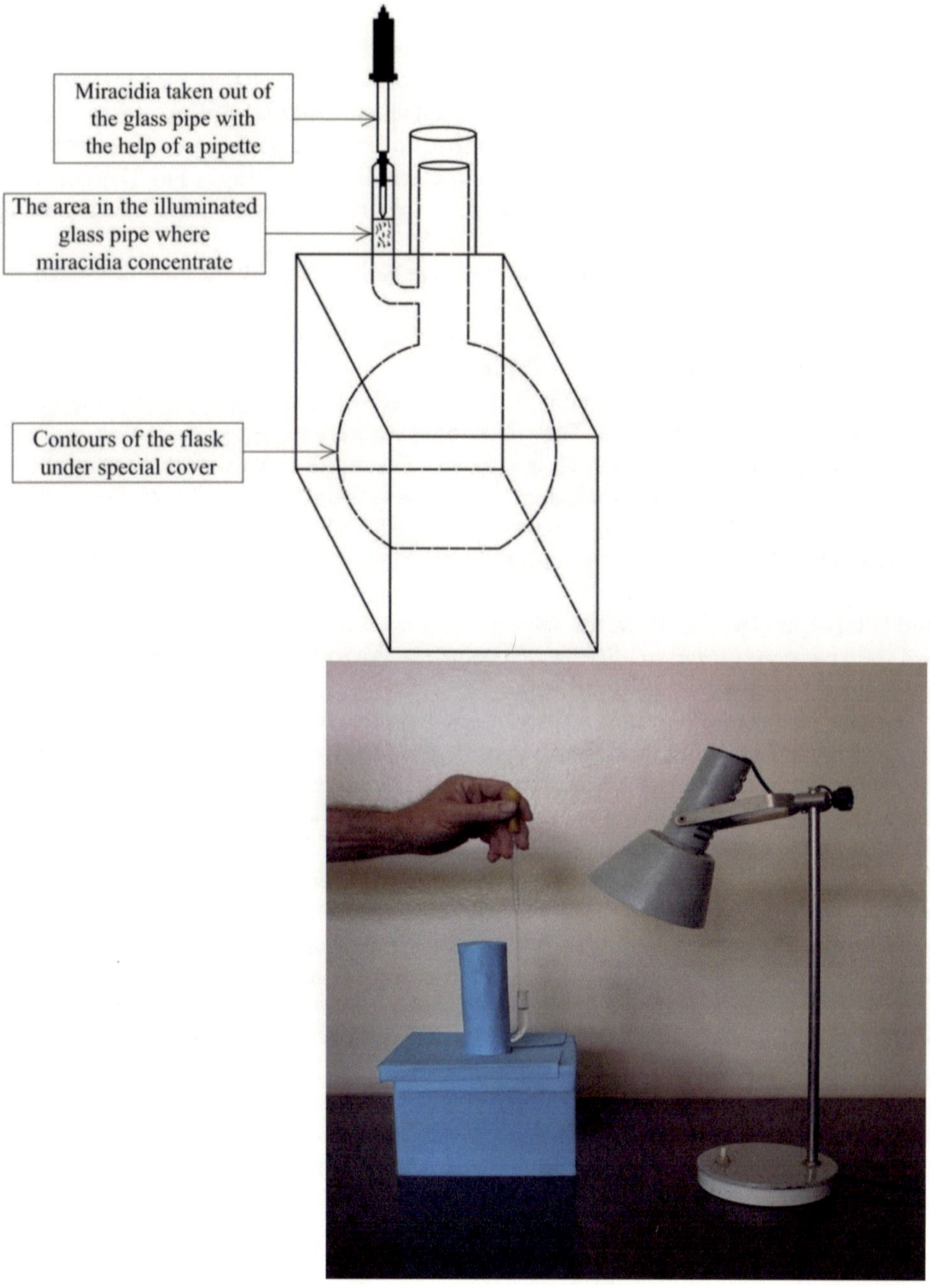

Figure 2.
The flask with a cover.

of neutral red following the methods of T.A. Ginetsinskaya (1987). The methods developed by K.V. Galaktionov and A.A. Dobrovolsky (1987) were used to examine the excretory system formula.

We infected animals with active cercariae of the same age, which were gathered 3–5 hours after they had left their intermediate host (the mollusc). We experimented on lambs, calves, young goats and young animals of other species. We infected each animal with cercariae (placing one of its ears into a vessel containing water with cercariae and heated to a temperature of 28–30°C, at intervals of 5, 10 and 30 minutes). We dissected the animals in 5, 10, 15, 20 and 30 days after they had been infected and studied the migratory routes of young maritae (schistosomula) of *Sch. turkestanicum*. We carried out the study using a phase-contrast microscope, inverted microscope CK2-TR (Olympus, Japan), microscope LOMO, cooling centrifuges TR7 (DuPont, USA), binocular ML-2200 (Olympus, Japan). The drawings were made using drawing apparatus PA – 4.

We used domestic and laboratory animals, as well as free-living molluscs—the intermediate hosts of the parasites under study—as a material for the field and laboratory research and experiments (**Table 1**). Additional researches (in 2000–2020) on animals were implemented as well (**Table 2**).

We studied the vertebrates using Skrjabin's method of complete and incomplete helminthological dissection [1]. The trematodes we were to study are known to concentrate in blood vessels, which is why we collected the parasites dissecting the vessels. It was a real problem to dissect the tiniest vessels (capillaries), and we decided not to. We did the following: first, pressing on the smallest vessels with the blunt end of a scalpel we brought the parasites into larger ones, which were then dissected and from which the trematodes were collected undamaged. The trematodes were then put into Petri dishes filled with water, where they stayed for 12–18 hours until they died, and then were preserved in a 70% spirit solution. We followed the common methods in studying the collected helminthes.

For the purpose to find out the rate of spontaneous infection with trematode cercariae and parthenitae in molluscs in various seasons, we carried out route research into the water bodies of the Amudarya and Syrdarya river basins. The stationary research was carried out in the water bodies of the middle and lower course of the Amudarya and the middle course of the Syrdarya.

The clinical presentations of schistosomiasis had been studying in 15 lambs and 30 rabbits, which had been artificially infected with *Schistosoma*. We used Sali's method to determine the quantity of erythrocytes and the methods of Hagedorn and Yensen to determine the leukogram, including blood corpuscle morphology, erythrocyte sedimentation rate, blood alkali reserve and sugar content. In the course of the general clinical observation of the lambs, we determined their general condition, temperature, pulse rate and respiration.

The crude protein in the blood serum was determined using refractometer, while individual protein fractions—using the electrophoresis method, on paper in apparatus EFA-1, after which elution and photometric measurements were carried out in photoelectric colorimeter FEK-M. The fractioning continued for 12 hours at a voltage of 200 V and a current strength of 0.3–0.4 ampere per a strip 1 cm wide. We used veronal buffer with pH 8.6 and an ionic strength of 0.05.

The strips were painted with bromophenol blue; the number of protein fractions was calculated for each experimental animal. The results of the first two series of research carried out before the lambs, and rabbits were infected with *Schistosoma* were regarded as initial. The results obtained in the course of the determination of protein fractions in the blood serum of the infected lambs and rabbits were compared with those obtained from the uninfected ones. Thus, we attempted to determine how the protein blood picture changes over the development of schistosomiasis.

The intestine, liver, pancreas, mesenteric lymph nodes, heart, kidneys, urine bladder, lungs and other organs of 10 sheep, 5 of which had been infected with *Schistosoma* naturally and 5 experimentally, were used as material for research of the

No.	Animal species	Quantity of specimens (vertebrates and invertebrates)
1	*Ovis aries*	4751
2	*Capra hircus*	139
3	*Bos taurus*	5293
4	*Camelus bactrianus*	16
5	*Equus caballus*	140
6	*Equus asinus*	17
7	*Sus scrofa* dom.	66
8	*Sus scrofa nigripes*	17
9	*Saiga tatarica*	33
10	*Felis ocreata* dom.	17
11	*Canis familiaris* dom.	21
12	*Oryctolagus cuniculus* dom.	156
13	*Citellus fulvus*	15
14	*Nesokia indica*	22
15	*Mus musculus*	38
16	*Anas platyrhynchos* dom.	64
17	*Anser anser* dom.	12
18	*Gallus gallus* dom.	46
19	*Lymnaea auricularia*	40,155
20	*L. corvus*	2923
21	*Larra truncatula*	4767
22	*L. stagnalis*	5127
23	*Planorbis planorbis*	3578
24	*Anisus spirorbis*	1476
25	*Anisus septemgyratus*	756
26	*Gyraulus albus*	3225
27	*G. ehrenbergi*	99
28	*Physa acuta*	6365
29	*Ph. fontinalis*	863

Table 1.
The species composition and quantity of studied animals.

pathomorphological changes in the organs. In addition, we studied these organs in 10 individuals of cattle infected sporadically with *Sch. turkestanicum*. The material was put into a 10% formalin solution, which was then poured into celloidin. The histological sections were dyed with haematoxylin-eosin following the method of Van Gieson.

We used over 50 specimens of molluscs *L. auricularia* infected with parthenitae and cercariae of *Sch. turkestanicum* to carry out the histological research. The digestive glands were cut out from live molluscs and put into 10% neutral formalin and 70%

Species	Researched, per.	Infected, %	
		Limits	M ± m
Cattle	2452	26.2–85.3	56.4 ± 6.8
Sheep	2175	20.0–46.0	34.1 ± 2.9
Goat	104	10.5–20.5	15.4 ± 1.1
Camel	26	5.2–15.2	10.1 ± 1.1
Horse	102	8.5–34.5	22.2 ± 3.0
Harc	36	5.5	
Bukhara deer	11	9.0	
Saiga	11	9.0	
Jeyran	13	7.6	

Table 2.
The rate of infection with mature schistosomes in certain animal species in Uzbekistan.

spirit. In order to carry out morphological estimation, we painted the sections with haematoxylin-eosin following the method of Van Gieson and Mallory [9–11].

Preparation of homogenate from the animal liver. In the experiments, we used 30 cattle specimens of the same age and sex, infected naturally with *Schistosoma*. These animals were selected based on the results of helminthoovoscopy. We took 10 specimens of uninfected animals from farms showing no signs of epidemy and used them as reference animals. The reference and experimental animals were slaughtered at the Khojeyli slaughterhouse in the Republic of Karakalpakstan. The cattle were dissected using Skrjabin's method of complete and incomplete helminthological dissection [1]. At the slaughterhouse, we cut several pieces from different parts of the liver and examined them. We put the pieces in a Thermos filled with ice.

To homogenise the tissue, we used a glass homogeniser with a ground surface. The tissue was homogenised for 20–30 seconds, in a tenfold solution of the emission environment, which contained 300 mM of sucrose and 10 mM of Tris of HCl buffer (pH –7.5).

Preparation of homogenate from trematode *Sch. turkestanicum*. After the animals had been slaughtered, trematodes *Sch. turkestanicum* were extracted from the veins of the mesentery and liver. The trematodes were washed in a separate container with physiological solution. After that, impurities were removed from them and they were delivered to a laboratory for homogenisation. The trematodes were homogenised in the same way as the cattle's liver was.

Preparation of homogenate from the liver of molluscs *L. auricularia.* About 10 to 15 mollusc specimens were put into separate vessels. We dissected the reference and experimental molluscs with a scalpel and cut out their livers. We determined the livers' mass and homogenised them using the method we used homogenising the liver of the cattle.

Extraction of lipids was implemented based on Folch's method [12]. We added 2 ml of a chloroform-methanol solution (2:1) to 0.2 ml of the reference sample (homogenate of the whole body of *Sch. turkestanicum* and the liver of molluscs and cattle), blended the mixture in a magnetic stirrer for 30 minutes, filtered it and put into a spinner flask, to which we added 1 ml of chloroform and 1 ml of distilled water. The mixture was blended carefully and spun at a speed of 3000 rpm for 10 minutes. The upper fraction was sucked out, and 0.5 ml of 10% KCl was added to the lower fraction. After being blended carefully, the mixture was again spun at a speed of

3000 rpm for 10 minutes. The upper water fraction was sucked out again, and the remaining substance was heated in a rotary evaporator until all the fluid evaporated and it became dry. Then, 0.2 ml of chloroform was added to the remaining substance; the substance was dried in gaseous nitrogen current and nitrogen atmosphere and was then kept in a freezer in a glass container with a tight stopper.

Fractioning of phospholipids using the thin-layer chromatography method. The thin-layer chromatography was carried out using silica gel and silica gel L5/40 micron manufactured by Chemapol (Czech Republic). Granulated silica gel was ground in a ball mill for 48 hours. To extract a narrow cut of sorbent with a particle size of 35–45 micron, we used the method described by A.D. Kargapolov (1981). The obtained adsorbent was kept in a hermetic container.

To determine the phosphor content, we used V. Vaskovsky's reagent [13].

Vaskovsky's reagent. A. Initial reagent: 400 mg of hydrochloric-acid hydrazine in 14 ml of 4H HCl was added to 10 g of sodium molybdate dissolved in 60 ml of 4H HCl. The mixture was heated in a boiling water bath for 20 minutes. Then, it was cooled and 14 ml of concentrated H_2SO_4 was added to it. Then, the volume of the mixture was increased to 100 ml. The reagent was kept in a dark glass container at an indoor temperature. B. Process solution. About 26 ml of H_2SO_4 was added to 5.5 ml of the initial reagent and the mixture was diluted with water until the volume reached 100 ml.

The method of one-dimensional thin-layer chromatography with a fixed adsorbent layer was used in the operation. In effort to prepare the sorptive substance, we shook hard a mixture of 3 g of silica gel and 0.17 g of gypsum in a flask. We then poured the mixture into a mortar and, grinding it carefully all the time, added 8 ml of distilled water slowly, in small portions. We blended silica gel with gypsum and water until they became a homogeneous. Then, we spread the mixture manually on a glass plate 9 cm by 12 cm in size, which had been carefully degreased before. Then, we dried it in a strictly vertical position in the air at an indoor temperature for 20–24 hours.

Just before use we activated the plates with silica gel at a temperature of 110°C for 1 hour. After the activation, a thin strip of silica gel, up to 0.2–0.3 cm wide, was removed from the edge of the plate along the whole perimeter. The reference sample solution was put onto a special spot, which had been marked in advance, with the help of a special glass capillary. After the sample was put, the plates were placed in a chromatographic chamber with a system of solvents, which had been saturated beforehand—petroleum ether (boiling temperature 40–60°C), diethyl ether and formic acid (at a volume ratio of 80:20:2)—to separate phospholipids from other lipids.

To fraction individual phospholipids, the plates with the samples were put into a chromatographic chamber with a system of solvents, which had been saturated beforehand—chloroform, methanol and 28% ammonia (at a volume ratio of 13:7:1). As the solvent front reached the required mark, the plates were taken out of the chamber and dried at an indoor temperature until no traces of solution remained. Then, the plates were placed in a chamber with iodine vapours. The spots with phospholipids became yellow-brown: they were pricked with a needle. The plates were then dried until no traces of iodine remained.

The phospholipid fractions were identified using standard phospholipid reference samples: phosphatidylcholine, phosphatidylethanolamine, cardiolipin, phosphatidyl inositol, phosphatidyl serine, phosphatidic acid and lysophosphatidylcholine. To do it, we spread the chloroform solution of the standard sample on individual plates and put it together with the plate, on which the studied phospholipid sample had been spread, in the chamber with a system of solvents. We established value R_f of individual phospholipid fractions on the reference and experimental plates with the range of phospholipids, following the formula given below [14]:

$$R_f = \frac{1}{m}$$

where 1 is the distance, the substance covers from the start to the centre of the spot; *m* is the distance covered by the mobile phase from the start to the front.

In an effort to determine the quantity of individual phospholipid fractions, phospholipids were scraped off the zone containing them together with silica gel into heat-resistant test tubes and added 72% per chloric acid (0.2 ml for large spots and 0.05 ml for smaller ones) [15]. The test tubes with the samples were put into a special thermostat (Kemcsotermosztat, made in Hungary) heated by electric power and kept them there at a temperature of 185–190°C for 20 minutes. After cooling, we added 1 ml of process solution into the test tubes and, stirring the substance carefully, kept in a boiling water bath for 15 minutes; then, we cooled it to an indoor temperature. We were separating the silica gel by spinning (2000 rpm for 10 minutes). We measured the optical absorption of supernates at a wavelength of 830 nm (red light filter) on spectrophotometer SPhM—26 in a cuvette with a layer 1 cm thick against the blank sample.

The protein content in the homogenates was determined following O. Lowry's method [16]. To do it, we added 9.95 ml of 0.1 NaOH to 0.05 ml of the studied solution, stirred the mixture and kept at an indoor temperature for 30 minutes. Then, we took 0.4 ml of the mixture and added 2.5 ml of reagent C and 10 minutes later we added 0.25 ml of solution E (Folin-Chokalteu reagent). Then, we stirred carefully the content of the test tube and in 30 minutes and measured it at 750 nm. We calculated the protein content according to a calibration schedule. Reagent C: we added 0.2 ml of solution B to 10 ml of solution A, stirred the mixture and kept it at an indoor temperature. Solution A: Na_2CO—a 2% solution in a 0.1 H NaOH. Solution *B:* $CuSO_45$ H_2O—a 0.5% solution in a 1% sodium citrate.

The gas chromatographic analysis of the fatty-acid composition of phospholipids. The hydrolysis and methylation of total phospholipids and their fractions. After the thin-layer chromatography had been carried out, we scraped the spots containing total phospholipids off into test tubes together with the silica gel and dissolved them in chloroform. Then, we filtered the mixture and evaporated the fluid from the solvent in a rotary evaporator until it became dry. The phospholipids were hydrolysed and methylated, following the method described by K.M. Sinyak et al. (1976). In this operation, we used glass test tubes with screwed-on stoppers and sealing gaskets of polytetrafluorethylene (Teflon).

The phospholipid extract concentrated to a drop was diluted by 5 ml of 1% sulphuric acid dissolved in methanol. The test tubes were then incubated in a water bath at a temperature of 80°C for 30 minutes. We added 2 ml of distilled water to the sample 3 minutes before the end of the incubation. After the incubation, we cooled the sample and extracted the methylated fatty acids of a mixture of hexane and ether (1:1) in three rounds. The mixed hexane-ether extract was concentrated through evaporation and diluted by 80–100 microlitres of a hexane-ether mixture (1:1).

The gas-liquid chromatographic measurements were carried out on chromatograph LChM-80 with a flame-ionisation detector, with the temperature of the thermostat being 180°C. The temperature of the evaporator and detector was 250°C. The dividing steel columns 3 m long and 3 mm across were filled with chromosorb W with 1.5% immobile phase s E-30 (INTERTON AW DMCS, 0.16–0.2 mm CHEMAPOL, Czech Republic). The recorder chart feed rate was 240 mm/h. The flow rate in the gas bearer of nitrogen was 30 ml/min, hydrogen—25 ml/min and air—300 ml/min. The amplifier sensitivity was 2×10^{-10}A. The peaks of the gas chromatogram were identified by comparing their duration time with the duration time of standard methylated fatty acids, such as myristinic, palmitic, stearic, oleic and arachidonic acids, as well as with literary data [17, 18].

The quantitative estimation of the chromatography was made by measuring the areas of the peaks of the components and determining their portion (in per cent) in the total amount of the areas of the peaks in the methylated derivatives of fatty acids (Stolyarov et al., 1988). The results of the experiments carried out in identical conditions were averaged according to a group of animals. The experimental data went through statistical processing, the certainty having been valued following Student's criterion, with the help of computer IBM PC/AT [19].

Author details

Djalaliddin A. Azimov[1], Bakhrom T. Norkobilov[2], Firuza D. Akramova[1], Ulugbek A. Shakarbaev [1] and Alisher A. Safarov[2]*

1 Institute of Zoology of the Academy of Sciences of the Republic of Uzbekistan, Tashkent, Uzbekistan

2 State Committee of Veterinary and Livestock Development of the Republic of Uzbekistan, Tashkent, Uzbekistan

*Address all correspondence to: safarov-alisher@mail.ru

References

[1] Skrjabin KI. The Methods of Complete Helminthological Dissection of Vertebrates, Including Human. Leningrad: Leningrad State University; 1928. p. 45

[2] Sukhachov VN, Dylis NV. The Programme and Methods of Biogeocenologic Research. Moscow: Nauka; 1966. p. 336

[3] Ginetsinskaya TA. Trematodes, their Life Cycles, Biology and Evolution. L: Nauka; 1968. p. 411

[4] Starobogatov YI. The Mollusc Fauna and Zoogeographical Regionalisation of the Continental water Bodies of the Earth. Leningrad: Science; 1970. p. 250

[5] Azimov DA. Tremadodes—Parasites of Animals and Human. Tashkent: Mehnat; 1986. p. 128

[6] Azimov DA, Akramova FD, Shakarbayev UA, Shakarboyev EB. Orientobildgarsii—Mammalian Trematodes. Tashkent: Fan; 2014. p. 224

[7] Shakarboev EB, Akramova FD, Golovanov VI, Azimov DA. Recommendations for the Prevention of Schistosomatosis in Livestock and Poultry. Tashkent: Fan; 2008. p. 27

[8] Ginetsinskaya TA, Dobrovosky AA. The new method of detection of trematode larvae's sensilla and the importance of these formations for the taxonomy. Uzbek Scientific and Research Institute. 1963;**151**(2):460-463

[9] Romeys B. Microscopic Technique. Moscow: Medicine; 1953. p. 708

[10] Merkulov GA. The Course of the Pathohistological Technique. Leningrad: Medicine; 1969. p. 422

[11] Volkova OV, Yeletsky YK. The Principles of Histology with the Histological Technique. Moscow: Medicine; 1971. p. 259

[12] Folch J, Lees M, Sloane-Stanley GH. A simple method for the isolation and purification of total lipids from animal tissues. The Journal of Biological Chemistry. 1957;**226**(1):497-509

[13] Vaskovsky VE, Kostetsky KG, Vasendin JM. A universal reagent for phospholipids analysis. Journal of Chromatography. 1975;**114**(1):645-647

[14] Akhmer AA, Kuznetsov AI. Thin-Layer Chromatography. M: Nauka; 1964. p. 176

[15] Bergelson LD. The Preparative Biochemistry of Lipids. Moscow: Mir; 1981. p. 329

[16] Lowry OH, Rosebrough HJ, Farr AL, Randall BJ. Protein measuremant with folin phenol reagent. The Journal of Biological Chemistry. 1951;**193**(1):265-275

[17] Keyts M. The Lipidology Technique. Moscow; 1975. p. 335

[18] Sinyak KM, Orgel MY, Kruk VI. The method of preparation of blood lipids for gas-chromatographic research. The Laboratorial Cause. 1976;**1**:37-47

[19] Marinichev AN, Turbovich ML, Zenkevich IG. Physicochemical Calculations on a Micro-IBM. L: Khimiya; 1990. p. 250

Chapter 4

The Morphology, Biology and Life Cycle of *Schistosoma Turkestanicum* Skrjabin, 1913

Djalaliddin A. Azimov, Firuza D. Akramova and Ulugbek A. Shakarbaev

Abstract

The chapter describes the features of the morphology, biology, and life cycle of *Schistosoma turkestanicum* Skrjabin, 1913. Synonyms of the above species and a list of definitive and intermediate hosts are presented in this chapter. This chapter also describes the localisation of the parasite, places of detection, morphometric parameters, and all phases of development of *Sch. turkestanicum*. The features of the development of parthenogenetic and dioecious generations of *Sch. turkestanicum* under experimental conditions are explained in the chapter. Emissions of cercariae were determined depending on photo-, thermo-, and geotaxis. The dependence of molluscs *Lymnaea auricularia* by larvae of *Sch. turkestanicum* on the seasons of the year has been established. A molecular genetic analysis of the population of mature schistosomes is presented. The morpho-biological features of *Sch. turkestanicum* and the circulation of invasions are substantiated on a large natural and experimental material.

Keywords: ontogeny, egg, miracidi, maternal, daughter sporocysts, cercariae, maritas, phototaxis, thermotaxis, geotaxis, molluscs *Lymnaea auricularia*

1. Introduction

Synonyms: *Ornitobilharzia turkestanica* (Skrjabin, 1913) Price, 1929; *Ornitobilharzia turkestanica* (Skrjabin, 1913), Dutt et Srivastava, 1955; *Orientobilharzia turkestanica* (Skrjabin, 1913), Dutt et Srivastava, 1955; *Ornitobilharzia turkestanica var. tuberculata* Bhalerao, 1932; *Ornitobilharzia cheni* Hsu et Yang, 1957.

Definitive hosts: *Bos taurus*, *Ovis aries*, *Capra hircus*, *Bubalus bubalus*, *Bibos indicus*, *Camelus dromedarius*, *Camelus bactrianus*, *Saiga tatarica*, *Alces alces*, *Capreolus cepreolus*, *Cervus elaphus, Equus caballus*, *Equus asinus*, *Equus* sp., *Felis ocreata* dom., *Sus scrofa*, *Rattus* sp. Experimentally infected animals—rabbit, white mouse, Indian gerbil and cavy.

Intermediate hosts: molluscs *Lymnaea* (=*Radix*): *L. tenera*, *L. auricularia*, *Lymnaea peregra* and *L. gedrosiana, L. ovata, L. luteola.*

Concentration: mesenteric arteries, the vessels of the liver, pancreas, intestine, sexual organs, urine bladder, gall bladder, heart and kidneys.

Discovery areas: Asia (Kazakhstan, Uzbekistan, Turkmenistan, Kyrgyzstan, Azerbaijan, Russia, Iraq, Iran, India, Pakistan, Mongolia, China, Nepal), Europe (France, Turkey and Hungary).

Description of the species (base on K.I. Skrjabin, in 1951; based on D.A.Azimov in 1986 with additions).

Male: the body is milky white, 8.6–15.0 mm long and 0.50–0.80 mm wide. The oral sucker is almost round, 0.30–0.36 mm in diameter, and the ventral one is slightly oblong, located 0.512–0.559 mm from the oral one, 0.36–0.40 mm in diameter. The oesophagus consists of two swellings; in front of the abdominal sucker, it is divided into two intestinal trunks, joining into an unpaired trunk at a distance of 2.10–2.58 mm from the tail end.

The testes are elongated and oval in shape, arranged in two rows between the intestinal trunks for 3.16–3.35 mm. The number of testes in most cases is 48–50, in some individuals more than 60. The gynaecophore channel is well-developed. The cuticle is without spines and tubercles (**Figure 1**).

Female: 6.5–8.5 mm long and 0.093–0.139 mm wide (always smaller than males). The suckers are rudimentary. The diameter of the oral sucker is 0.036–0.048 mm. The abdominal sucker lies at a distance of 0.206–0.216 mm from the

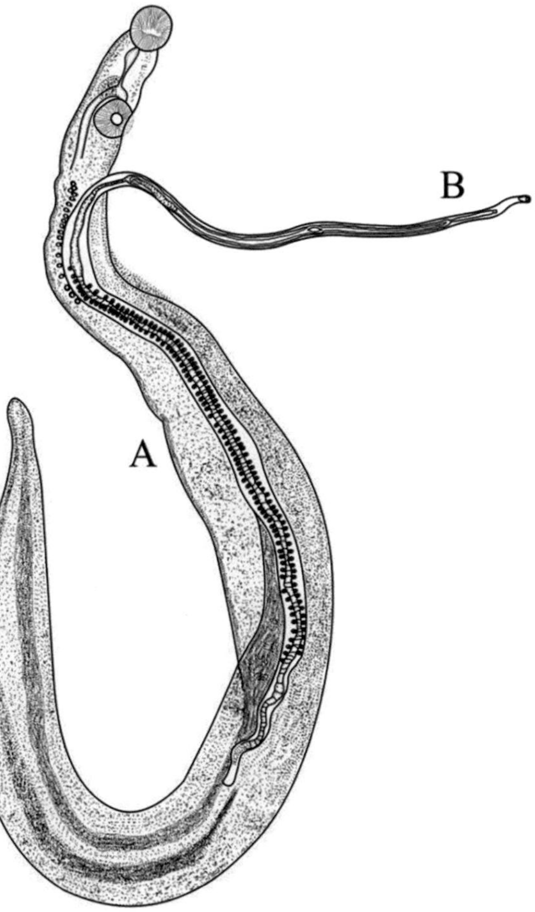

Figure 1.
Schistosoma turkestanicum Skrjabin, 1913. The general view of the male (A) and female (B) (by Azimov, 1975).

mouth, 0.028–0.038 mm in length and 0.0186 mm in width. The oesophagus is simple, at the anterior edge of the abdominal sucker it is divided into two intestinal trunks, which join into an unpaired trunk in front of the yolks. The ovary has the form of a spiral-rounded tube, located along the longitudinal axis of the body; dimensions—0.380 × 0.046 and 0.420 × 0.046 mm. The rounded yolks lie on the sides of the unpaired intestinal trunk. In the uterus, one egg is elongated and oval in shape and has one spike on each of the poles. Egg length is 0.078–0.084 mm and width is 0.024–0.027 mm. The length of the pointed spike is 0.008–0.009 mm (**Figures 1** and 2).

The development cycle of *Sch. turkestanicum* has been studied [1–14]. The intermediate hosts of this trematode in different regions of Asia and Europe are various species and subspecies of freshwater molluscs of the genus *Lymnaea* (=*Radix*). Parthenites and cercariae develop in the body of molluscs. Mature cercariae that have emerged from the host molluscs enter the final host, where the maritogony ends with the formation of male and female flukes. The first mature eggs containing miracidia are found in the faeces of sheep, goats and cattle 40–55 days after infection [15–17].

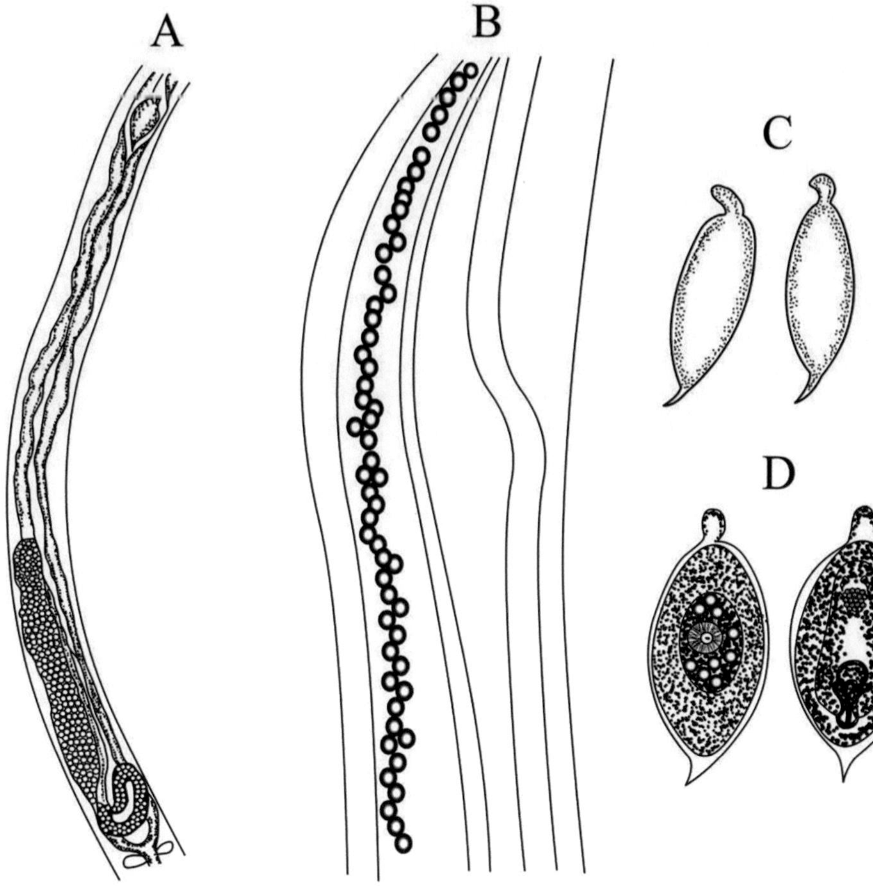

Figure 2.
Schistosoma turkestanicum Skrjabin, 1913: A—female's part of the body with the uterus and ovary; B—male's part of the body testes; C—eggs; and D—stages of eggs' development (by Azimov, 1975).

Literature[1]: Skrjabin, 1951; Azimov, 1975, 1986; Azimov et al., 1965–2012; Zakhryalov, 1975; Shakarboyev, 1996, 2009; Gorokhov, 1963; Chauhan et al., 1973; Massoud, 1973, 1974; Lien et al., 1975; Sahba, Malek, 1979; Tang et al., 1983; Liu et al., 1987; Athari et al., 1990, 2006; Wang et al., 2000, 2002, 2009; Lockyer et al., 2003; Farahnak, Essalat, 2003; Li et al., 2008; Qiu et al., 2008; Majoros et al., 2010.

Below is given the description of the morphology and biology of all the development stages of *Sch. turkestanicum*, based on the results of enormous field and experimental research carried out in various biogeocoenoses of Uzbekistan.

2. The egg and miracidium

Based on our observations it was determined that, as they develop, *Sch. turkestanicum* maritae penetrate into the tiniest veins adjacent to the wall of the intestine and lay the eggs, which are not yet fully developed, in the lumina of the small vessels. The laid eggs are oval and elongated and have one thorn on each pole. One of the thorns has the form of a slightly bent appendix, and the other—an appendage, which seems to be tightened at the connection with the egg body. The length of the eggs is 0.074–0.082 mm, and the width is 0.021–0.026 mm. The length of the sharp thorn is 0.006–0.008 mm. Going out of the uterus, the egg contains a fertilised ovum surrounded by vitelline cells.

Further development and formation of miracidium in the egg occur in the host tissues (**Figure 3**).

As *Sch. turkestanicum* eggs develop their morphology variation. First, the embryo cell divides consecutively into two, four, eight and sixteen cells. Then, the embryo goes through the morula and blastula stages to become a miracidium in the end. As the embryo develops, the yolk cells, which serve as nutrients for the future miracidium, begin to decrease in number until they disappear completely, when the miracidium becomes fully developed.

In the course of embryogenesis, the eggs of *Sch. turkestanicum* go through various metric changes together with morphological ones. Thus, the size of the freshly laid egg is 0.074–0.082 mm, and by the time, it is ready to go out of the host's organism, it has reached 0.13–0.14 mm in length. As the eggs run along the vessels and inside the tissues of the host, they develop to be absolutely mature, with a mobile, fully grown miracidium, at the moment they leave the host's organism. It is one of the forms of biological adaptation characteristic of *Sch. turkestanicum* and the whole blood fluke suborder at the early stages of their ontogenesis. In our opinion, embryogenesis of this type is highly progressive and testifies to the perfect adaptation of trematodes from the schistosome suborder to life in the closed systems of their hosts.

Schistosoma's eggs taken from the hosts' faeces are oval and elongated, with one thorn on each of the poles. One of the thorns is usually sharp and the other blunt. The colour of the eggs is ash grey. The egg contains a mobile, fully developed miracidium covered with dense cilia.

The size of a mature egg is 0.13–0.14 × 0.042–0.064 mm. The length of the sharp thorn is 0.008 mm.

[1] The 1906–1950 literary data are generalised in K.I. Skrjabin's monograph "Trematodes of animals and humans" ("Трематоды животных и человека" (1951. Vol.5); the 1951–1975 data are given in D. A. Azimov's book 'Schistosomes of animals and humans' ("Шистозоматиды животных и человека" (1975). Therefore, we refer to literary sources not indicated in the abovementioned works.

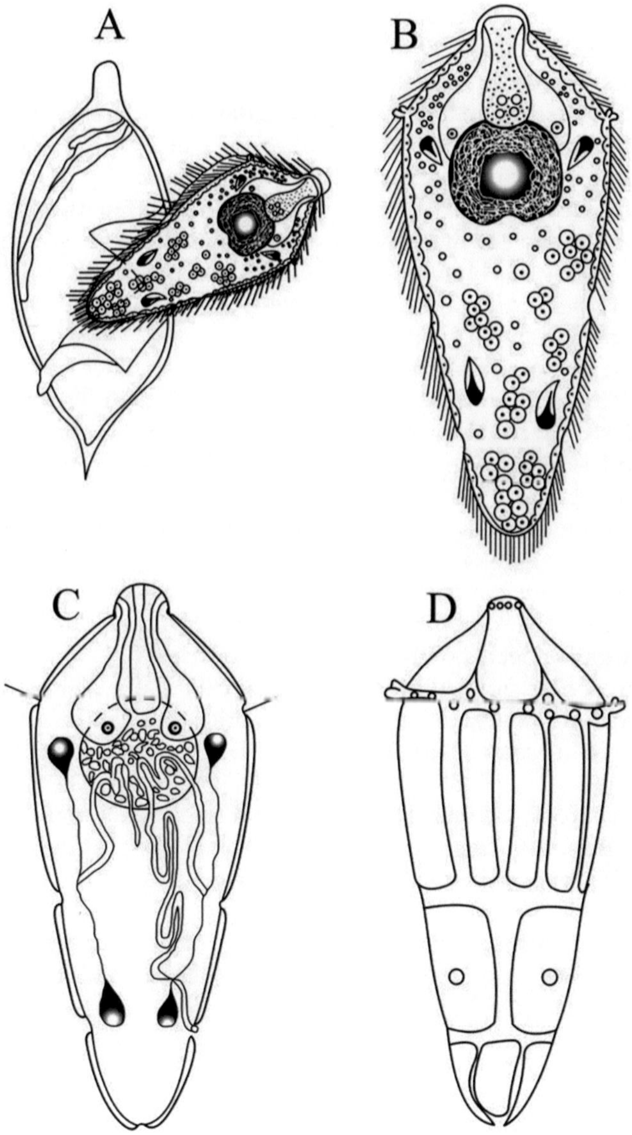

Figure 3.
Schistosoma turkestanicum Skrjabin, 1913: A—A miracidium emerging from the egg; B, C—Fragments of organs; and D—Disposition of the epithelial plates and sensilla.

3. The miracidium in the egg and its leaving it

It was identified that almost all of the eggs of *Sch. turkestanicum* found in the hosts' faeces had miracidia in them. When the egg containing developed miracidium contacts water, the movement of the miracidium and the cilia can be noticed. The miracidia become more active in the egg.

The miracidium uses a proboscis to adhere firmly to the inner surface of the eggshell. It makes pendular movements, which become more active in course of time. Then, the miracidium begins to spin fast around the longitudinal axis of the egg, and later the rotation becomes more active, but this time around the transversal axis. The egg always breaks in the lateral wall; the break has never been observed in the lateral wall near the thorn. The miracidium's exit from the egg is conditioned by the miracidium's movements and, probably, the increase of pressure inside the egg. The external environmental factors play an important part in the miracidium's exit from the egg. The optimal temperature is +13–28°C and pH –6-7. Light is also an absolutely necessary condition. The exit process continues 30–60 seconds.

The form of a live miracidium's body and the ratio of its length to its width may vary according to its movement. However, when immobile or fixed, miracidia have an elongated body ending in a blunt tail. The rear end is narrower than the front one.

Miracidium is the first larval stage in *Schistosoma*'s complex life cycle. Its biological goal is to infect the intermediate host.

Except for the proboscis, the miracidium's body is covered with cilia, which rests on the epithelial plates. The number of epithelial plates is 22, their disposition following the formula 6:9:4:3. The intestine is a short and relatively thick tube. The intestine tube is flanked on both sides by two penetration glands. They are longer than the intestine and their rear ends bordering on the nerve knot. The nervous system is a rather thick spherical mass occupying roughly the central position in the miracidium's body.

A number of nerve trunks formed of nerve fibres sprout from it.

The excretory system consists of two pairs of flame cells and their tubes. One of the pairs is located in the front part of the body, and the other is in the rear part. The flame cells are interconnected with the help of capillaries.

The embryo cells are situated behind the nerve cells and occupy a large space inside the miracidium's body. In most cases, they are located in the rear part of the body and gathered in groups. These cells are rather large and spherical, with a clearly visible nucleus.

The miracidia of *Sch. turkestanicum* have a structure similar to the structures of other miracidia from the Schistosomatidae family. It means that the miracidia from one phylogenetic group of *Schistosomatidae trematodes* are uniform in structure.

Studying the morphology of the coat of the parasite's miracidia we discovered varying numbers of epidermal plates, up to 20–22 in some larval specimens. However, very few miracidia had 21 epidermal plates. Usually, developed *Sch. turkestanicum* miracidia in most cases had 22 plates—6:9:4:3.

A miracidium that has just emerged from the egg moves very fast along a straight line. It may change direction very suddenly, going down deep underwater or approaching its surface. We noted that these miracidia do not stop moving until they naturally die. During all this time, they search for their intermediate host.

Taxes play an important part in miracidia's life. Interacting, different taxes propel miracidia to the part of the water body inhabited by molluscs, which are the intermediate hosts of this trematode species [18]. According to T.A. Ginetsinskaya, taxis determine miracidia's motion relative to sources of light, gravity and chemical stimuli.

We established that miracidia of *Sch. turkestanicum* are characterised by prophototropism and ageotropism. These data conform to the literary sources [19]. Miracidia are very active when light is diffused, concentrating in the superficial layers of water. Therefore, miracidia's taxes should be regarded as an adaptive capacity developed in the course of evolution and ensuring contact between the larvae and their intermediate host.

T.A. Ginetsinskaya (1968) maintains that miracidia are usually ageotropic, and their taxis in most cases are connected directly to the biology of the mollusc species, which is the intermediate host of this very miracidia species. The combination of photo- and geotropism is the principal condition that allows a miracidium to get into this or that part of the body of water. The author considers that the biological meaning of the combination of tropism types is based on the ecology of molluscs, miracidia's intermediate hosts, which coincides with our opinion. So, the mollusc *Lymnaea auricularia*, *Sch. turkestanicum* intermediate host, inhabits clean and warm bodies of water with slimy bottoms and much vegetation [20]. In addition, ear molluscs can be encountered in small swamps, little shallow canals near pastures, puddles and floodplain lakes in steppes [21]. The molluscs are active on warm sunny days, concentrated on the surface of the water bodies.

The prophototropism and ageotropism propel the miracidia of this *Schistosoma* to the illuminated surface of the water body, where it contacts the ear mollusc, its intermediate host.

When they meet a mollusc, miracidia begin to chase it, alternately approaching and moving away from their host. Miracidia usually do not stay long at molluscs as they are not their intermediate hosts (families Planorbidae, Physidae), while seeing *L. auricularia* they move fast towards them and attack them, trying to penetrate into their body. Attacking the molluscs miracidia contact the latter's body and seem to stick to it. After that we watched miracidia penetrating into their intermediate host through its coat, which usually took 20 to 30 minutes. We observed that *Sch. turkestanicum* miracidia can live up to 24 hours at a temperature of 28–30°C.

4. The development of parthenitae and cercariae in the intermediate host

We recorded that *L. auricularia* [6, 22–24], a freshwater mollusc species widely distributed in Uzbekistan, were naturally infected with *Sch. turkestanicum* parthenitae and cercariae.

We infected artificially molluscs aged 15–20 days bred in the laboratory. We infected them individually, keeping them in small saltcellars together with 1–2 miracidia. In some cases, we infected molluscs by bringing a few miracidia to a vessel containing a certain number of molluscs, with the number of miracidia not exceeding four specimens per mollusc. The infected molluscs were kept in cuvettes at a temperature of 28–32°C. Further, the molluscs were dissected regularly and inspected for *Schistosoma* parthenitae.

Penetrating into the host's body the miracidia undergo regressive metamorphosis and turn into a mother sporocyst. The latter is a bag filled with reproductive products. It propagates parthenogenetically, producing daughter sporocysts—specimens of the next generation.

Mother sporocysts become fully developed by the 7th or 8th day, containing mobile sporocysts. The mother sporocyst is 0.252–0.609 mm long and 0.035–0.231 mm wide. The embryo cells are spherical in form and have a core. Sometimes embryo cells are elongated and are located within the mother sporocyst. The daughter sporocysts form on the embryo cells of the mother sporocyst. They become mobile on the 8th or 9th day after they penetrated into the mollusc, tear the membrane of the mother sporocyst and move freely within the host's organs, mainly the liver. The daughter sporocyst also has the form of an elongated bag containing a number of embryo cells. The size of daughter sporocysts varies. On the 12th–15th day after the infection of the molluscs, the daughter sporocysts were 0.096–0.483 mm long and 0.021–0.053 mm wide. Later the length of the daughter sporocyst increases and it gives birth to a number of cercaria embryos. The developed cercariae leave the daughter sporocyst through the end puerperal opening on the 22nd–25th day (**Figure 4**).

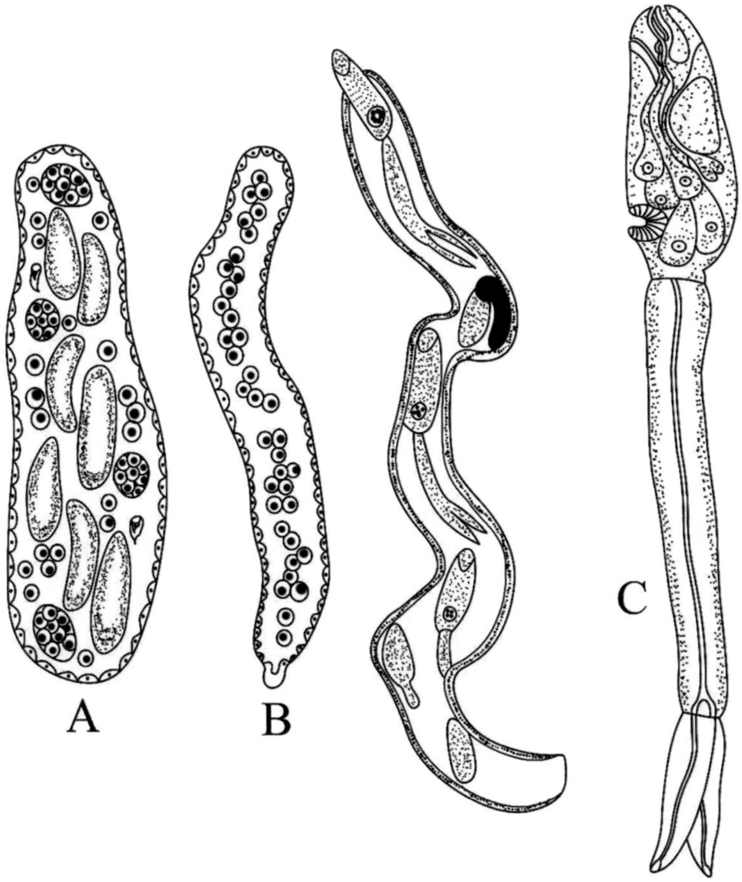

Figure 4.
Schistosoma turkestanicum Skrjabin, 1913: A—mother sporocyst; B—daughter sporocyst; and C—Cercaria [25].

The cercariae that have left the mollusc's organism have an original tail branching at the tip. They belong to a pharyngeal brevifurcocercariae without eyespots.

Given below are the morphological parameters of *Sch. turkestanicum* cercariae, which we determined in the course of our research (**Table 1**). The cercariae's tegument is covered by numerous visible thorns. Their size decreases from the head towards the tail.

Part of the body	Cercariae	
	Died naturally	Dyed with carmine acetate
Body: length and width	0.160–0.189 0.048–0.064	0.120–0.146 0.043–0.060
Front organ	0.058–0.063	0.049–0.056
Ventral sucker	0.050–0.059	0.042–0.051
Tail: length and width	0.193–0.231 0.024–0.028	0.042–0.051 0.101–0.196
Tailfurcae: length	0.080–0.096	0.021–0.024

Table 1.
The size of Sch. turkestanicum cercariae (mm), n = 100.

The cercaria has an oval body, 0.160–0.189 mm long and 0.048–0.064 mm wide. The tail stem is cylindrical, narrowing slightly towards the end. The length of the tail is 0.193–0.231 and the width is 0.024 mm. The tail furcae are 0.080–0.096 mm in length.

The front organ is highly muscular, pear-shaped or oval, 0.058–0.063 mm long and 0.050–0.054 mm wide. It is located right at the front of the body.

The penetration glands consist of five pairs of cells. Their ducts are directed forward, towards the front organ. The ducts are very long, occupying almost the whole of the cercaria's inner surface.

The ventral sucker is well-developed and is situated in the rear part of the body. Its size is 0.050–0.059 mm.

The digestive system. The mouth opening is located ventrally, leading to the oesophagus connected to the intestine. The digestive system has the form of a thin-walled tube widening at the end. The structure of the intestinal tube variates depending on the position of the body.

The nervous system consists of nerve cells, which form concentrations interconnected with thin fibres. The nerve knot is located in the front part of the body.

The excretory system consists of five pairs of vibratile cells and pipes linking them. The excretory duct opens at the end of the tail branching. The vibratile cells are dislocated following the formula 2 [(2) + (2) + (1)] = 10.

The system of sexual organs usually is not differentiated. They have the form of concentrations of spherical cells located behind the ventral sucker.

The sensory apparatus of the *Sch. turkestanicum* cercaria consists of the following complexes: the end, ventral, dorsal, lateral and furcal complexes. The end complex consists of 36 sensilla concentrated around the front organ. Sensillae—sensitive endings of the nervous system of trematode larvae—have long attracted the attention of parasitologists.

Up to nowadays, sensillae have been identified in the cercariae of various groups of trematodes, including Schistosomatidae. In some representatives of the genera *Schistosoma, Schistosomatium* and *Ornithobilharzia* cercariae chaetotaxy (topography and number of sensillae on the body) have been studied using a variety of techniques. After the introduction of new methods into the laboratory practice of helminthological studies, such as staining sensillae and especially various modifications of the method of impregnating sensillae with a solution of silver nitric acid (Wagner, 1961), a new stage in the study of the sensory apparatus of cercariae began. There were special works on the study of cercariae chaetotaxy in some species of cercariae from the family Schistosomatidae. The authors noted that certain types of studied cercariae are characterised by a specific structure and topography of sensillae, which is important from the diagnostic viewpoint. Information about the sensory organs of *Sch. turkestanicum* cercariae is practically scarce. For this reason, we studied the chaetotaxy of *Sch. turkestanicum* cercariae produced by *Limnaea (=Radix) auricularia* molluscs from bodies of water in the lower reaches of the Amu-Darya river.

In our effort to identify the sensillae of *Sch. turkestanicum* cercariae, we used the method of impregnating with a 1% solution of silver nitric acid (Wagner, 1961). A total of 25–30 cercariae extracted from a mollusc were placed in water on a piece of glass with a hole. Then, the water was sucked off with a thin pipette, 2–3 drops of silver nitric acid were added and the hole with cercariae in the reagent was covered with black paper. The cercariae were thus kept for 3–5 minutes. Then, the silver solution was sucked out with a pipette and the cercariae were thoroughly washed. This procedure was repeated up to 10 times with distilled water. After that, the cercariae were transferred to bright daylight for 5–10 minutes. Then, they were put on a slide in a drop of clarifier consisting of lactic acid and glycerol in equal parts and covered with a cover glass.

The study of the sensory apparatus of the *Sch. turkestanicum* cercariae showed that the sensilla located on the body of the cercariae are characterised by stable constancy both in number and in topography. Sensilla are found both on the body and on the tail and are located symmetrically, although they show minor individual variations. The total number of sensilla is about 90. Most of them are concentrated on the body and tail trunk. The general pattern of the arrangement of sensilla is shown in **Figure 5**.

As shown in **Figure 2**, the ventral complex consists of 38 sensillae, the dorsal 26 and the lateral 22. The total number of sensillae is 86. For individual cercariae, the number of sensillae reached 90–94.

The location of the sensillae on certain parts of the *Sch. turkestanicum* cercariae was quite stable. So, the body identified—42, senzill on caudal trunk—34 and furko—10. A large part of the symmetrically located senzill marked on the body and tail of the barrel.

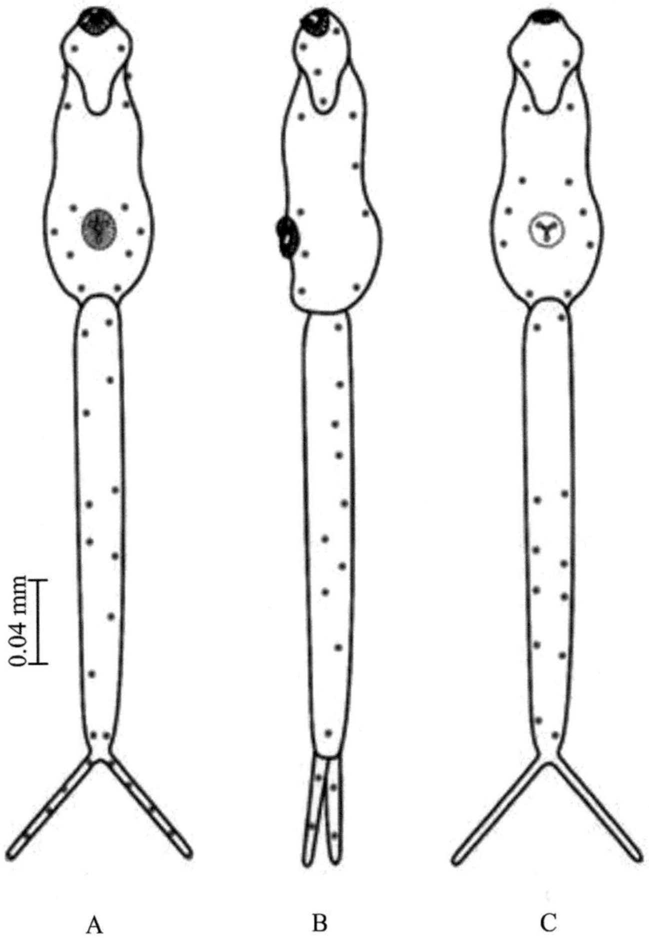

Figure 5.
Schistosoma turkestanicum Skrjabin, 1913. Sensor device for cercariae Sensilla's disposition: A–ventral complex; B–lateral complex; C–dorsal complex.

The implemented study showed that the sensory apparatus of the *Sch. turkestanicum* cercariae consisting of several complexes is characterised by sufficient stability in the number and order of the sensors, which is an additional feature for differentiating species of the Schistosoma genus, which is consistent with the views of the authors.[1]

The obtained results about the structure of the sensory device of the *Sch. turkestanicum* cercariae also confirm the known data of literature in chaetotaxy other types of schistosomes about the possibility of their use for species identification representatives of cercariae of trematodes of the Schistosomatidae family.

Live organisms, regardless of their morphological structure, are characterised by cycles that can also be recorded in helminths.

Helminths' biorhythms are conditioned by the relations with their hosts, as well as the biotic and abiotic factors of the external environment.

Based on the specificity of helminths' biology, we think it expedient to differentiate the biorhythmic parameters in the intermediate host's organism. We have carried out some research into the daily rhythms of *Schistosoma* cercariae's emission from the molluscs, their intermediate hosts.

In order to study the biological rhythms of the cercariae's emission, we used freshwater molluscs *Lymnaea auricularia* from the water bodies of the Syrdarya and Amudarya river basins infected with trematode larvae.

We have registered the dynamics of the daily rhythms of the cercariae's emission and their dependence on the illumination, temperature and reaction of the environment. To do it, we put molluscs infected with relevant cercaria species into separate glasses, three specimens into each one. The volume of water in each glass was 250 ml, with pH 7–8 and a temperature of 19–28.5°C. All the glasses were equally illuminated. Once in 1 hour, we registered the number of cercariae coming out of the molluscs for 24 hours.

The total number of *Sch. turkestanicum* cercariae specimens that went out of the molluscs in 24 hours was 3755. In the afternoon (between 12.00 and 6.00 p.m.), the larvae proved to be the most active, with 716–1110 specimens having left their hosts' bodies in this period. At the same time, no cercariae went out in the evening hours (**Figure 6**).

In the nighttime, the cercariae's emission came to a complete stop. When the temperature was lowered to 16–17°C the number of cercariae coming out of the molluscs decreased greatly, and no cercariae left the molluscs when the temperature dropped to 10–12°C. The optimal recorded temperature for cercariae's coming out of molluscs was 22.5–24.5°C.

The results of the research allow us to suppose that the daily rhythms of *Sch. turkestanicum* cercariae's emission from the molluscs depend on environmental factors. These factors activate or slow down the emission of cercariae from the mollusc, as well as its other vital functions [27].

The daily rhythm of cercariae's emission breaks, if the illumination schedule changes. So, when the molluscs were in permanent darkness with the optimal temperature and environment reaction, no cercariae left their hosts. In the nighttime, when the molluscs were illuminated with artificial light, cercariae left their hosts; however, their number was small.

The daily rhythms of cercariae's emission from their intermediate hosts and various emission conditions typical of each of the species play an important part in the formation of trematodes' life cycles and their circulation in biocoenoses. The adaptation to these conditions has developed in the course of the evolution of the parasite-host relations and aims at ensuring maximal contact between cercariae and their definitive host, in which the subsequent ontogenetic stages take place.

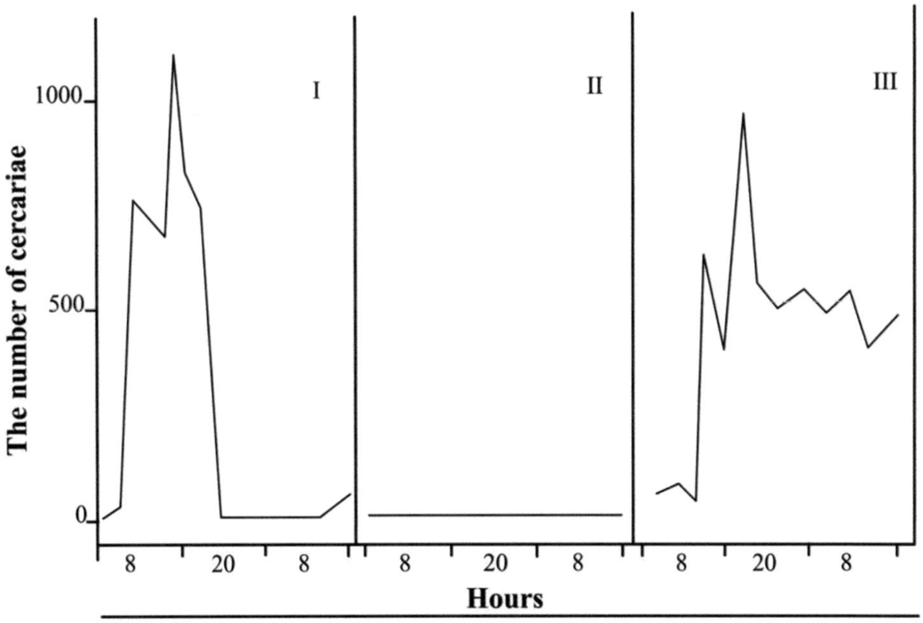

Figure 6.
Daily rhythm of Sch. turkestanicum cercariae's emission: I—at natural alternation of day and night; II—in permanent darkness; and III—in permanent illumination [26].

According to our observations, the cercariae's emission activity actually coincides in time with the utmost activity of their definitive host and it should be regarded as trematodes' adaptation to the host's ecology and behaviour.

Therefore, the synchronous development of the helminths and their hosts' vital functions finally ensures the circulation of infection in biocoenoses. However, a biocoenosis's components control strictly this process.

Cercariae of *Sch. turkestanicum* are characterised by prophototropism, prothermotropism and ageotropism, which was established by experiments.

Standard test tubes 15 cm long and 1.5 cm in diameter were used to determine *Schistosoma* cercariae's geotropism. The experiments were carried out at a temperature of 24.5°C. We poured water with the cercariae into a glass test tube and shook it carefully to distribute the larvae equally throughout the height of the test tube. The test tube was placed vertically on special support and illuminated with natural light. Within 3–5 minutes, the cercariae went up to the surface of the water. This proved the cercariae's ageotropism (**Figure** 7).

To determine the cercariae's phototropism, we put trematode larvae that had just left their host into a test tube with water and stirred the content to spread the larvae equally throughout the height of the tube. Then, we placed the test tube in a horizontal position and darkened a part of it with a black paper bag, after which, within 6–8 minutes, the cercariae moved to concentrate in the illuminated part of the test tube.

Then, we removed the paper bag from the darkened part and placed it in the part that had earlier been illuminated. In this case, the cercariae reacted quickly and moved actively to the illuminated part of the test tube. In another experiment, we darkened the test tube on both sides, leaving a gap 2 cm wide in the middle of the test tube, along its circumference. In this case, again, the cercariae concentrated in the illuminated part of the test tube. Therefore, *Schistosoma* cercariae are characterised by express prophototropism.

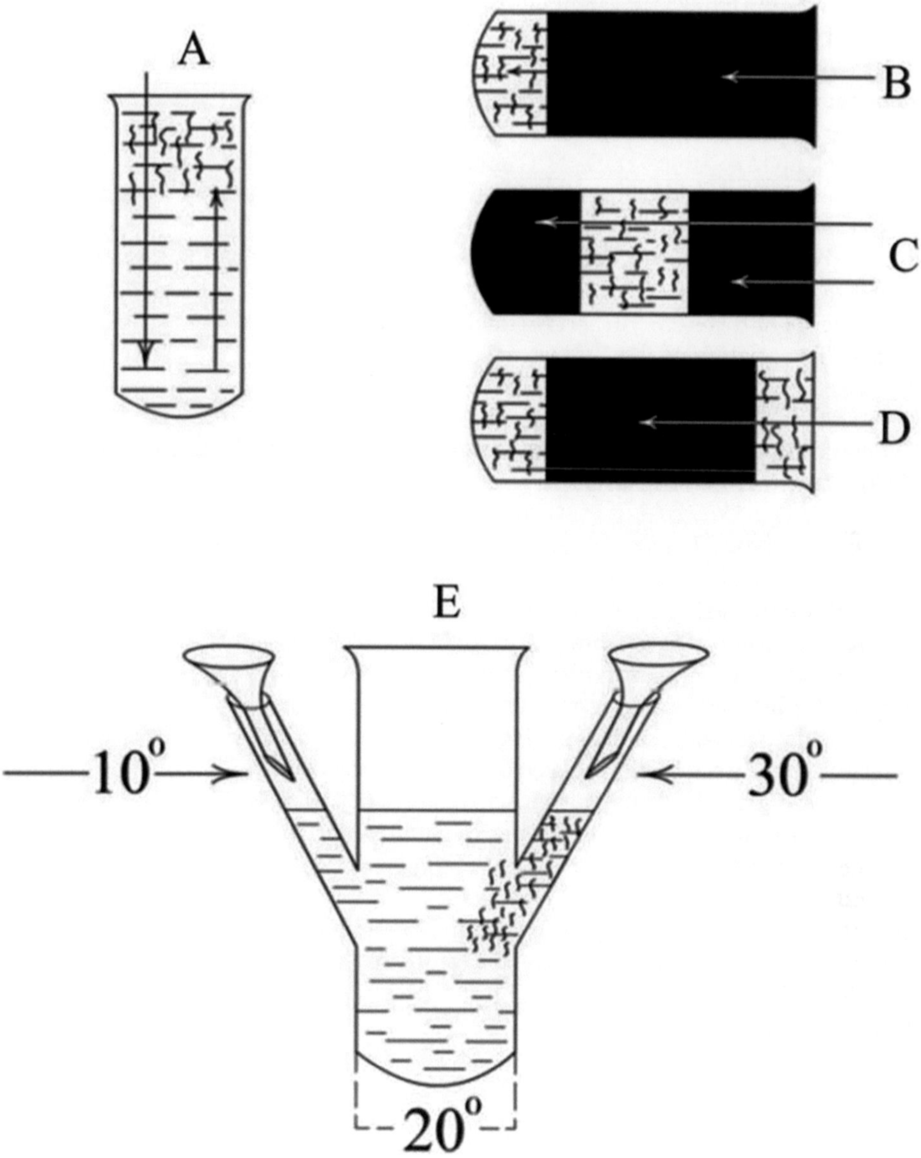

Figure 7.
The taxis of the Schistosoma turkestanicum cercariae: A–negative geo; B, C, D, E—positive figure and thermo—Taxises (by Azimov and others, 2019).

In effort to determine the cercariae's thermotropism we used a vessel with two lateral pipes with an inner diameter of 2 cm made especially for this purpose. We filled the horizontal part of the vessel with water with cercariae of this species, the temperature of which was 19–20°C. After that, we filled one of the pipes with 10°C water and the other with water heated to 30°C. In 5–10 minutes, all the cercariae moved to the pipe with warm water, concentrating in its upper layers. In 15–20 minutes, the cercariae got into the second pipe, too, as the diffusion in the vessel had brought to the equalisation of the temperature. This testifies to prothermotropism in cercariae of *Sch. turkestanicum*. The types of tropism described above ensure the cercariae's contact with their definitive hosts.

Cercariae's life expectancy depends on a number of factors, as well as on the amount of glycogen in their tissues [18].

Cercariae's activity occupies an important place in their life process and depends on temperature and illumination. In our experiments (with a participation of at least 100 cercariae in each experiment), the cercariae lived up to 72 hours at a temperature of 10–18°C, up to 48 hours at 25–28°C and 37 hours at 28–30°C.

Comparing nucleotide sequences 18Sin the Uzbek population of *Sch. turkestanicum* we established that they differed in only one nucleotide.

Thus, the analysis of nucleotide sequences in the well-known *Sch. turkestanicum* populations demonstrates that this trematode species do not vary throughout its range. The slight difference in certain nucleotide sequences can be ascribed to the intraspecific variation of this *Schistosoma*.

5. The ecology of molluscs *Lymnaea auricularia*, intermediate hosts of *Schistosoma turkestanicum*

Stationary research into molluscs was carried out in bodies of water in the lower stretches of the Amudarya and Syrdarya Rivers. In other regions of Uzbekistan, molluscs were studied using transect surveys.

Snail *L. auricularia* is a common species in the biocoenoses of various types of bodies of water and, certainly, plays an active part in the circulation of elements and the spread of helminths among animals and humans. This is why researchers from various fields of science, such as zoologists, helminthologists and hydrobiologists, are interested to study the biology and ecology of *L. auricularia.*

L. auricularia are known to be hermaphrodites (Zhadin, 1952). They are egg-laying animals. According to our survey, the mollusc lays fertilised eggs in clutches of 6 to 40 eggs. The clutches are lanceolate. The eggs are regularly oval, 0.87–0.88 mm long and 0.72–0.74 mm wide. The clutches are attached to various substrates. Most often the substrate is plants or shells from the same mollusc species. In the laboratory, the clutches of *L. auricularia* can often be found on the surface of a crystalliser and on the moist surface of plants (mulberry, grapevine and reed leaves). Each egg contains one or sometimes two embryos.

We established that embryogenesis lasts 27–28 days at a temperature of 10–12°C, 21–24 days at 14–17°C and 7–8 days at 20–30°C.

As they hatch, young snails develop very rapidly and begin laying eggs 25–33 days after hatching.

The shell of the newly hatched mollusc ranges between 0.84 and 0.86 mm in length (0.85 mm on average) (**Figure 8**).

The mollusc's active postembryonic development continues from the very first days after hatching until they reach the age of 25–35 days, when the length of their shells is 13.0–16.0 mm and the width 8.0–9.05 mm. After that the molluscs' growth slows, which is associated with the breeding period (as well as environmental conditions). The snails reach their maximum size by the end of the year, when their shell is 24.0–25.5 mm long and 16.0–18.0 mm wide.

In natural conditions, the pond snails feed primarily on aquatic plants. In the laboratory, we used mulberry and grapevine leaves and semolina, which we ground to a fine substance before bringing to the aquarium. The snails were developing very rapidly in the laboratory. For one-year *L. auricularia* in the water bodies of Uzbekistan produce 3–4 generations. According to the field research, this mollusc occurs

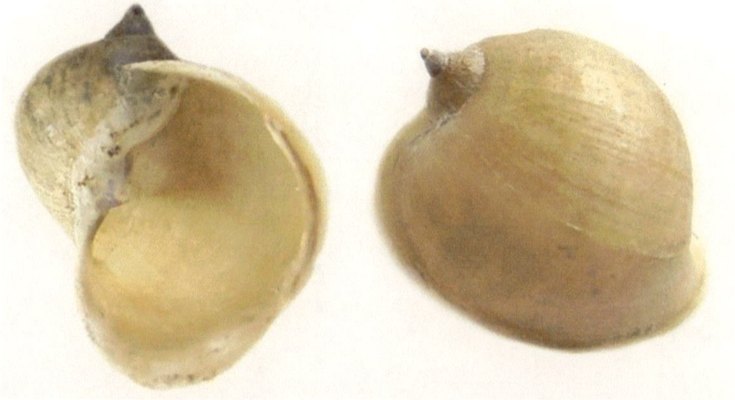

Figure 8.
Mollusc Lymnaea auricularia, the intermediate host of Schistosoma turkestanicum.

throughout Uzbekistan in all freshwater bodies with an environment suitable for its development. *L. auricularia* prefers shallow well-warmed bodies of water with silty bottoms. It often occurs on algae-covered stones near the waterside, in lakes, swamps, canals near pastures, ponds and flood water. *L. auricularia* is most abundant in small canals near pastures and lakes, where we recorded 100–200 individuals per 1 m^2.

L. auricularia lives on the surface of silt in various bodies of water. The abundance of this mollusc is extremely high near the waterside.

The pond snails are particularly active in the warm season, between May and September. The abundance of *L. auricularia* was 200–300 individuals per 1 m^2 in water heated to 25–30°C, while in October, when the water temperature lowered to 10.0–10.3°C, the abundance dropped to 1–7 individuals per 1 m^2.

The density of an *L. auricularia* population is dependent directly on environmental conditions and, according to our observations, varies between 1 and 300 individuals per 1 m^2 of biotope. This species occurs mostly in spring and summer, when the temperature of the air is 20°C and higher, while in autumn and winter they, probably, hide within silt, under the surface of the ground, near plant roots, and remain in hibernation [21].

The rate of infection with cercariae of *Schistosoma* in molluscs *L. auricularia* was established only in the water bodies of the north-western (Republic of Karakalpakstan, Khorezm province) and north-eastern (Syrdarya, Tashkent and Jizzakh provinces) parts of Uzbekistan [6, 22, 25, 28].

In the north-western part of Uzbekistan, 87 of the 115 studied bodies of water proved infected with schistosomiasis. In the north-eastern part, only 9 of the 45 studied bodies of water turned out to be infected with this *Schistosoma*.

The dynamics of the infection with *Schistosoma* cercairase in molluscs *L. auricularia* were studied in certain bodies of water in the lower course of the Amudarya and middle course of the Syrdarya Rivers.

We established that the rate of infection with parthenitae and cercariae of this trematode varied greatly (**Figure 9**). In the north-west of Uzbekistan, the infection rate was 0.3–45%, and in the north-eastern part of the country – 0.4–5.0%.

The dynamics of the infection with *Schistosoma* cercariae in molluscs *L. auricularia* depends directly on the environmental conditions, primarily, on temperature. The earliest mature cercariae develop in molluscs in June (0.5–1.0%), the latest in July (15–45%). By autumn the infection rate drops considerably.

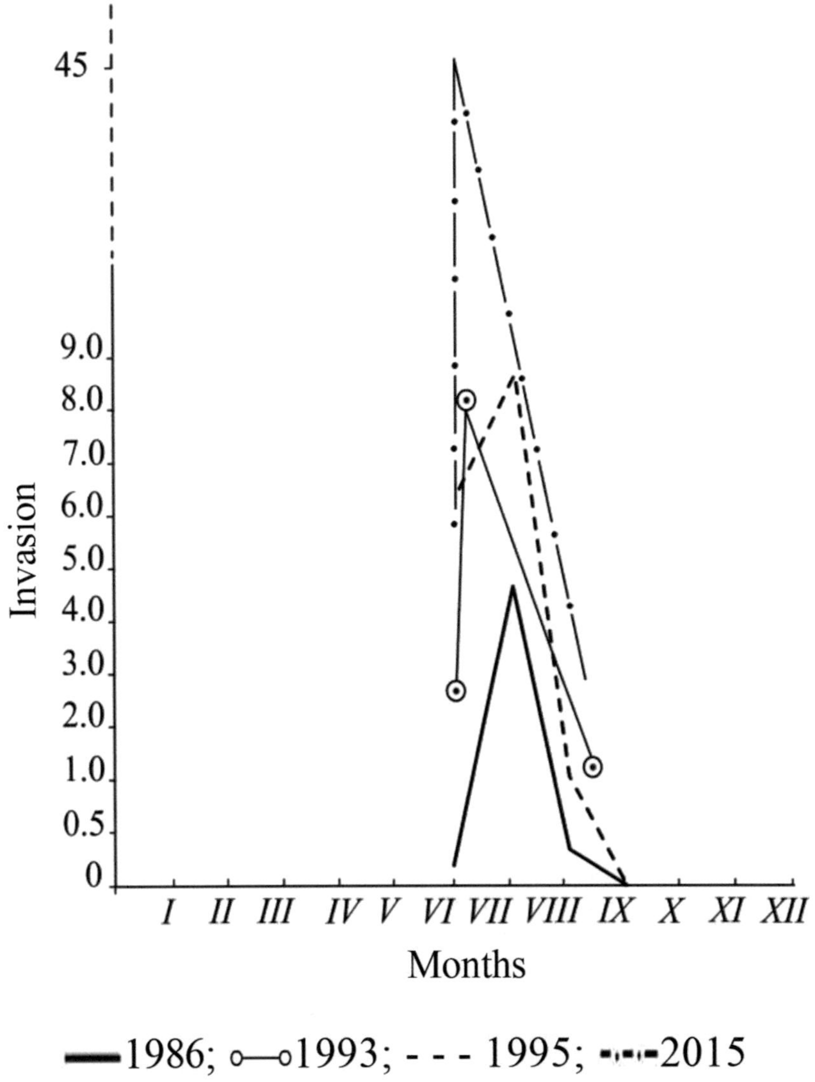

Figure 9.
Dynamics of the infection with larvae of Schistosoma turkestanicum in Lymnaea auricularia in various years: — 1986; o—o 1993; - - - 1995; -.-.- 2015.

In the course of observation in a natural biotope in one of the water bodies in the Dautkul lake system we noted that the number of cercariae emerging from one individual of pond snail during the day reached 7435, with 4235 larvae leaving the host's organism between 8 a.m. and 12 noon, 110 larvae between 1 p.m. and 4 p.m. and 2990 between 5 p.m. and 8 p.m.

Thus, we are absolutely certain that *L. auricularia* in the north-western and north-eastern parts of Uzbekistan—regions problematic in terms of schistosomiasis—produce stable cercariae populations. Letting out huge numbers of cercariae, they ensure dense concentrations of infectious organisms in the parts of water bodies next to the waterside, which leads to a high level of infection in *Schistosoma*'s definitive hosts. Moreover, migrating from one body of water to another the infected molluscs help the infection spread among susceptible animals.

6. The development of *Schistosoma* maritae in the organism of the definitive host

Local and foreign researchers established that cercariae of *Sch. turkestanicum* can penetrate into the definitive host's organism both percutaneously and perorally [1, 3, 7, 29].

The experiments were carried out on white mice, rabbits and lambs. Cercariae from experimentally and sporadically infected molluscs *L. auricularia* were used to infect the test animals. The cercariae were brought inside the animals percutaneously, perorally (with drinking water) and intraperitoneally.

In order to infect the animals perorally we used pipettes to give them water with cercariae. To infect them percutaneously we fixed them immobile and kept one of their ears in a glass with water infected with cercariae for 3–30 minutes. After that, we counted the remaining cercariae to established the number of parasites that have penetrated into the animals. The rabbits were infected intraperitoneally by syringing water with cercariae into their abdominal cavity. All the animals infected in various ways were dissected after definite periods of time. To find trematodes we studied the animals using the complete helminthological dissection method.

We found out the ways of infection by the areas in the animals' organisms in which the parasites were discovered. We estimated the survival rate of the cercariae that had penetrated into the animals' organisms by comparing the number of trematodes that had developed in the bodies with the initial number.

The white mice and rabbits were infected with trematodes both percutaneously and perorally. The infection rate varied between 30.0% and 100.0% according to the infection method used.

The percutaneous method resulted in a 100.0% infection rate in the rabbits and sheep and 46.6% in the white mice. The use of the peroral method brought to the infection rate of 30.0% in the mice, 50.0% in the rabbits and 61.5% in the sheep. Zero infection rate was recorded when the animals were infected intraperitoneally.

Thus, the principal ways of infection with *Schistosoma* are percutaneous and peroral, which conforms with the literary data [1, 3, 7].

The time required for cercariae of *Sch. turkestanicum* to penetrate into the definitive host's body and their survival rate also deserve attention. To establish it we carried out experiments on rabbits and white mice.

The experimental data demonstrate that *Schistosoma* cercariae penetrate very quickly into the organism of a definitive host. A 5–10-minute contact with the body of a host (a mouse or rabbit) is enough for the larva to penetrate into it. Our research conforms to data from other scientists [3], with the only difference being that in our experiments cercariae penetrated even faster.

The cercariae that have penetrated into the host's organism turn into schistosomula (**Figure 10**).

We establish that schistosomula's acclimatisation rate is relatively high, ranging between 11.2 and 4 3% (average 29.7%) when the animals were infected percutaneously and between 0.6 and 15.2% (average 9.6%), when they were infected perorally.

In our opinion, the difference between the acclimatisation rate in schistosomula taken percutaneously and the one in those taken perorally arises from the fact that only part of the larvae taken by mouth cling to the upper portions of the digestive tract and the rest get into the stomach, where, affected by the gastric juice, die, while those penetrating the host percutaneously go directly to the blood system and migrate to the place they stay in and develop.

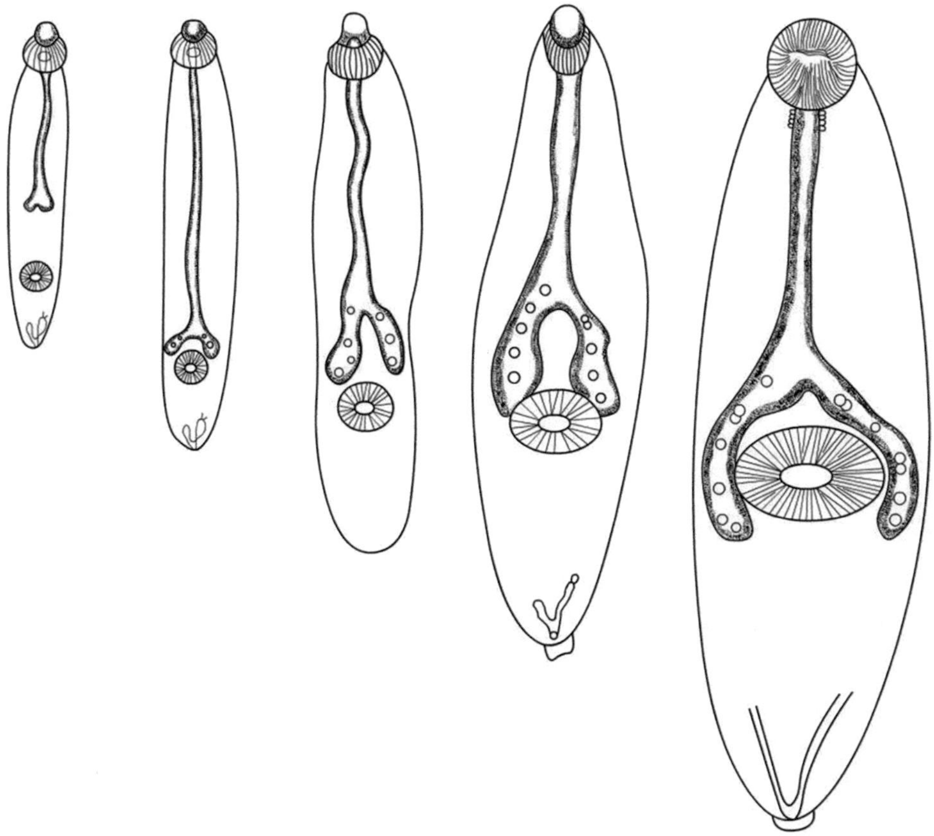

Figure 10.
The development of Schistosoma turkestanicum Skrjabin, 1913 in the organism of a definitive host: Developing trematodes [26].

Therefore, cercariae of *Sch. turkestanicum* get into their host by penetrating actively through its uninjured skin. Thus, they avoid contacting the secretion and juices of their host's digestive tract, which are very harmful to them. Having acquired the ability to penetrate actively into the organism of their definitive host, larvae of this species, as well as all other trematodes parasitising the blood vessels of vertebrates, changed their morphology and biology.

The cercariae actually became "aggressive", which gives them a lot of advantage in penetrating into the host's organism and speeds up the development of this trematode in the wild.

After the penetration of the cercaria into the host's organism, its ontogenesis undergoes considerable qualitative changes.

The first changes of the trematode in the organism of the definitive host (sheep) occur two days after the infection when the parasites are found in the lung swabs. In this period the schistosomula still have the penetration organs. The parasite's intestine also changes somewhat. Its distal end widens and the first signs of branching into two stems appear. The size of the trematode is 0.160–0.190 × 0.048 mm.

Three days later trematodes 0.190 × 0.050 mm in size were found in the swabs of the lungs and liver. The penetration glands were clearly visible. The intestine was elongated; it contained dark bodies and its distal end reached the ventral sucker. In four days, the parasites were found in the liver, lungs, heart and mesenteric arteries. Their size and morphology were identical to those described above. The trematodes found in five days after the infection in the liver, lungs, heart and mesenteric arteries had the following size: 0.210 × 0.057 mm, 0.200 × 0.055 mm and 0.220 × 0.057 mm. The trematodes still had penetration glands, but they were poorly visible. The intestine's size was larger than usual. Its distal end was also elongated.

Eight days later the schistosomula were found only in the liver and mesenteric arteries. No penetration glands were found. The size was 0.300x0.055 and 0.300 × 0.060 mm, respectively (**Figure 10**). On the 10th day, the trematodes were found only in the liver and the mesenteric arteries. The size of the parasites was 0.342 × 0.065 mm. The mouth sucker was well seen. The intestinal branches went around the ventral sucker. In 15 days, the parasites were 0.680–0.860 mm long and 0.060–0.070 mm wide (average 0.770 × 0.065 mm). The intestinal branches did not unite into a common tube. Rudiments of periesophageal glands appeared. The trematodes were not yet differentiated sexually. They began to divide into males and females on the 18th–20th day. The males were thicker than the females but much shorter. The males were 1.640–1.740 mm long and 0.089–0.102 mm wide. The suckers were well-developed. The intestinal branches united into a single tube at the rear of the body. The females were longer than the males and were 1.400–1.840 mm long and

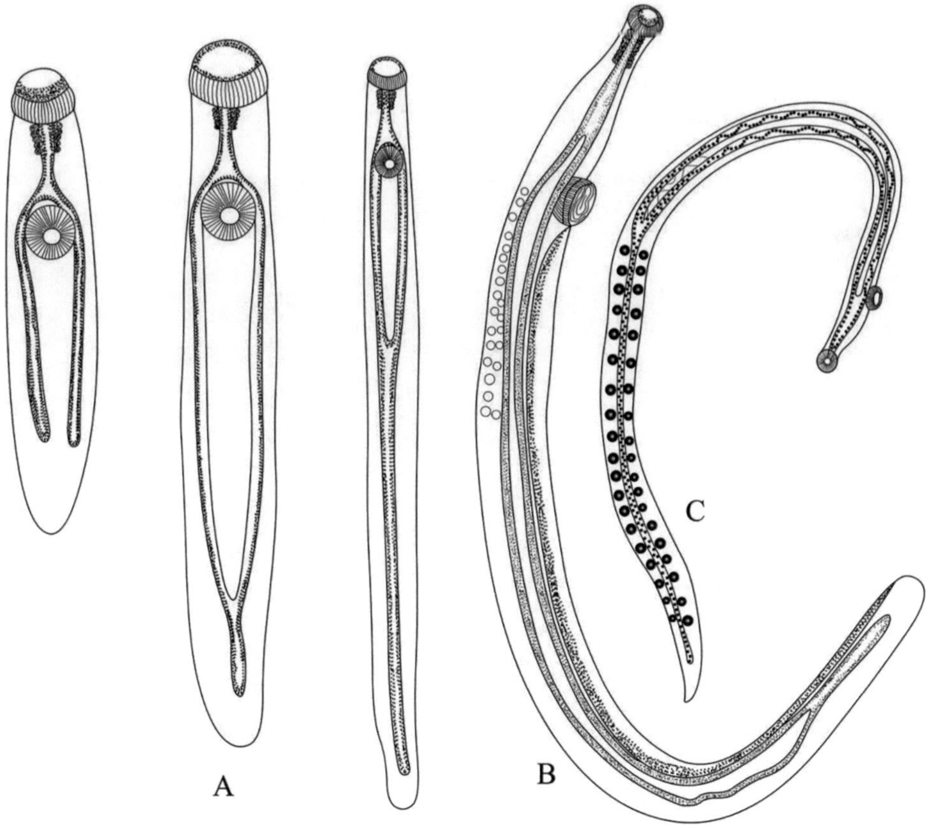

Figure 11.
Development of Schistosoma turkestanicum Skrjabin, 1913 in the organism of a definitive host: A—developing trematodes; B—male; and C—female [26].

0.065–0.076 mm wide. The intestinal tubes united into an unpaired tube in the front part of the body. The cuticle of both the males and females is smooth.

In 25 days, the males and females become the same size. The males continue to grow fast and finally become larger than the females. The length of the males is 2.854–2.944 mm and the width is 0.102–0.128 mm. The gynecophoral canal is well-seen. The suckers are well-developed. The contours of the seminal gland are now visible behind the ventral sucker. The paired intestinal tube is long. The cuticle is smooth. The female is 2.560–2.854 mm long and 0.065–0.089 mm wide. The mouth sucker is not seen well. The female now has the uterus and the spiral ovary. The paired intestinal tube is short. The intestinal tubes unite into one right behind the seminal gland and continue to the end of the body. The vitelline glands, which have not yet formed properly, are located on the sides of the unpaired intestinal tube (**Figure 11**).

In 32–35 days after the infection, the trematodes were mainly paired both in the mesentery and in the liver. Both the males and females were quite developed (**Figure 12**).

In the course of implemented research was identified that *Schistosoma turkestanicum* becomes mature in the organism of the definitive host (rabbits, sheep) in 32–35 and 32–40 days, respectively. The first mature eggs appear in the faces of sheep in 50–55 days.

We established that maritae concentrate mainly in the vessels of the mesentery, liver, pancreas and under the mucous membrane of the intestine. If an animal was heavily infected with *Schistosoma*, the trematodes may be found in the veins of the host's other organs, which conforms with the data given by MacHattie (1936), Zakhryalov (1969), Panin and others, (1968).

The long life of the parasite in the organism of the definitive host is one of the factors ensuring the mutual adaptability and stability of the "parasite-host" system.

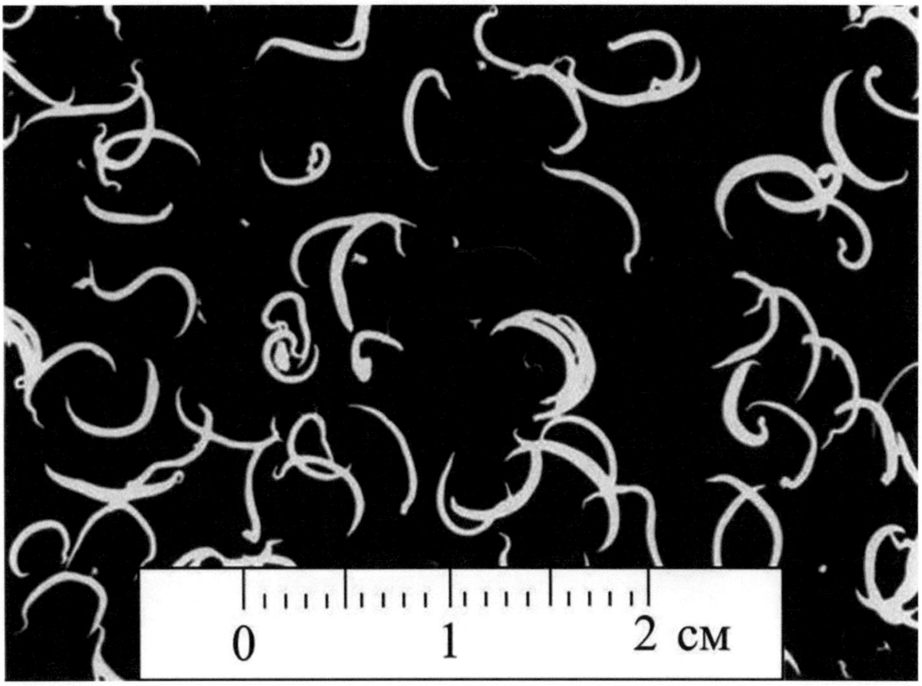

Figure 12.
Schistosoma turkestanicum Skrjabin, 1913: Mature trematodes found in the mesenteric artery of sheep [26].

In the course of our observations, we established that *Sch. turkestanicum* can remain alive in the organism of the definitive host for quite a long period. So, *Schistosomes* live for over 10 years in cattle, 8 years in sheep and 3.5 years in rabbits.

The lifespan of *Schistosoma* in the organism of the host, probably, depends on the latter's reactivity and the form of relations in the "parasite-host" system, which has formed in the course of their evolution [30].

Author details

Djalaliddin A. Azimov, Firuza D. Akramova and Ulugbek A. Shakarbaev
Institute of Zoology of the Academy of Sciences of the Republic of Uzbekistan, Tashkent, Uzbekistan

*Address all correspondence to: safarov-alisher@mail.ru

References

[1] Mac Hattie C. A preliminary note on the life history of *Schistosoma turkestanicum* Skrjabin, 1913. Transactions of the Royal Society of Tropical Medicine and Hygiene. 1936;**30**:115-124

[2] Zakhryalov YN. The intermediate host of *Ornithobilharzia turkestanica* (Skrjabin, 1913) in the Far East. The Materials of a Scientific Conference. 1965;**Part. 1**:90-95

[3] Zakhryalov YN. The ways of the infction of the definitive host with *Ornithobilharzia turkestanica*. The Materials of a Scientific Conference. 1968;**Part 1**:118-122

[4] Zakhryalov YN. On the biology of Ornithobilharzia turkestanica (Skrjabin, 1913) in the Far East. In: Natural Diseases and the Questions of Parasitology in the Republics of Central Asia and Kazakhstan. Vol. 5. Almaty: Donish; 1969. pp. 155-158

[5] Zakhryalov YN. *Orientobilharzia turkestanica* (Skrjabin, 1913) Dutt and Srivastava, 1955 in the Far East: The abstract of a doctoral thesis. Alma-Ata: Institute of Zoology. 1975:43

[6] Azimov DA. The issues of the epizootology of orientobilharziasis in ruminants. Veterinariya. 1966;**11**:50-52

[7] Panin VY, Lavrov LI, Uvaliyeva KK. The study of the life cycle of *Ornithobilharzia turkestanica* (Skrjabin, 1913). In: The Materials of the Conference Dedicated to the Memory of N. V. Badanin. Tashkent: Fan; 1968. pp. 246-247

[8] Kumar V. Studies on snail hosts of *Orientobilharzia turkestanicum* (Skrjabin, 1913) Dutt et Srivastava, 1955 (Schistosomatidae: Trematoda). Annales de la Société Belge de Médecine Tropicale. 1973;**53**(1):17-23

[9] Massoud J. Studies on the Schistosomes of domestic animals in Iran. I. Observations on *Ornithobilharzia turkestanica* (Skrjabin, 1913) in Khuzestan. Journal of Helminthology. 1973;**67**(2):165-180

[10] Massoud J. Observations on Lymnaea gedrosiana, the intermediate host of *Ornithobilharzia turkestanica* in Khurzestan, Iran. Journal of Helminthology. 1974;**48**(2):133-138

[11] Tang C, Tang Z, Cao H, Tang L, Yu CQQ, Lu H. Research into *Orientobilharzia turkestanica* parasitizing sheep in the eastern part of an autonomous district in Inner Mongolia. Dunu syuebao, Acta Zoologica Sinica. 1983;**29**(3):249-255

[12] Dutt SC, Srivastava HD. Studies on the life history of *Orientobilharzia turkestanica* (Skrjabin, 1913) Dutt and Srivastava, 1955. Current Science. 1964;**22**(24):752-753

[13] Amid A, Gohar S, Rosnami M. Dermination of definitive and intermediate hosts of cercarial dermatitis-producing agents in northern Iran //. Archives of Iranian Medicine. 2006;**9**(1):11-15

[14] Majoros G, Dán A, Erdélyi K. A natural focus of the blood fluke *Orientobilharzia turkestanica* (Skrjabin, 1913) (Trematoda: Schistosomatidae) in red deer (*Cervus elaphus*) in Hungery. Veterinary Parasitology. 2010;**170**(3-4):218-223

[15] Azimov DA. *Ornithobilharzia turkestanica* (Skrjabin, 1913) in sheep and cattle. In: A Treatise Issued by

Uzbek Scientific and Research Institute. Veterinary. Vol. 17. Tashkent; 1965. pp. 9-10

[16] Shakarboyev EB. The Ecological and Functional Interrelations of *Orientobilharzia Turkestanica* (Skrjabin, 1913)—*Bos taurus* Linnaeus, 1758 in the Parasite-Host System: A PhD Thesis in Biology. Tashkent: Institute of Zoology. 1996. p. 134

[17] Azimov DA, Akramova FD, Shakarbayev UA, Shakarboyev EB. Orientobildgarsii—Mammalian Trematodes. Tashkent: Fan; 2014. p. 224

[18] Ginetsinskaya TA. Trematodes, their Life Cycles, Biology and Evolution. L: Nauka; 1968. p. 411

[19] Lavrov LI. The copper, iron, proteins and tryptophan contents in the tissues of *Ornithobilharzia*. In: The Materials for the Republican Seminar-Conference for the Control of Parasitic and Non-contagious Diseases Agricultural Animals. Alma-Ata; 1974. pp. 184-187

[20] Zhadin VI. Molluscs in the Fresh and Brackish Waters of the USSR. Guides into the Fauna of the USSR. Moscow: Science, 1952. p. 374

[21] Azimov DA. Freshwater mollusc Radix auricularia as the intermediate host of *Ornithobilharzia turkestanica* in Uzbekistan. The Uzbek Biological journal. 1968;**4**:42-44

[22] Azimov DA. The biology of *Ornithobilharzia turkestanica* in Uzbekistan. Report by the Academy of Sciences. 1969;**7**:52-53

[23] Azimov DA. On the relation of trematode *Ornithobilharzia turkestanica* (Skrjabin, 1913) to specific hosts. The materials of a scientific conference. Moscow. 1971;**23**:6-10

[24] Azimov DA. The biology of trematode *Trichobilharzia ocellata* in Uzbekistan (Schistosomatata: Ornithobilharziidae). The Uzbek Biological Journal. Vol. 3. Tashkent: Фан. 1977. pp. 44-46

[25] Azimov DA. The ecological principals of the protection of the environment from helminths. In: The Protection of the Animal World of Uzbekistan. Tashkent: Fan; 1975. pp. 45-48

[26] Azimov DA, Akramova FD, Shakarboyev EB, Norqobilov BT, Shakarbayev UA, Sayitqulov BS. Schistosomiasis of Animals. Tashkent: Fan; 2019. p. 320

[27] Markevich PA, Chernogorenko MI. The daiy rhythm of cercariae's emission as a result of their relation with the hosts and the latter's dependence on the abiotic factors of the environment. The all-USSR Symposium for the Diseases and Parasites of Aquatic Invertebrates. Leningrad: Science; 1976. pp. 47-43

[28] Azimov DA, Dadayev S. The daily biological rhythms of cercariae's emission. Reports by the Academy of Sciences. 1977;**5**:67-69

[29] Azimov DA, Nurmukhamedov KN. Orientobilharziasis in ruminants. The Agriculture of Uzbekistan. 1967;**7**:56

[30] Azimov DA. On the habitats of trematodes from the genus *Orientobilharzia*. In: The Uzbek Biological Journal. Vol. 3. Tashkent: Фан. 1978. pp. 44-46

Chapter 5

Interrelations of *Schistosoma Turkestanicum* Skrjabin, 1913 in the System of the "Parasite-Host"

Djalaliddin A. Azimov, Firuza D. Akramova, Alisher A. Safarov and Erkin B. Shakarboev

Abstract

The chapter presents experimental data on the relationship of *Schistosoma turkestanicum* in the host parasite system of interconnected groups, alternating parasitic and free-living states of this trematode, where the physiological and biochemical aspects of parasite-host relationships in animals with schistosomiasis are considered. Particular attention is paid to the population structure of *Sch. turkestanicum*, mature forms that parasitise in the blood vessels of mammals and larval forms in aquatic molluscs. The implementation of the adaptive-compensatory mechanisms of the parasite and the host ensures the functioning of the parasitic system. The dynamism of the system depends on a complex of factors of exogenous and endogenous origin. The life of free-living populations (miracidia and cercariae) of *Sch. turkestanicum* is suppressed by unfavourable abiotic environmental factors. The number of parasitic populations depends on endogenous (biotic) factors. This is evidenced by the results of experimental studies—physiological and biochemical changes in the blood, protein fractions and histostructure of individual organs of infected animals, which are detailed in the text of the book.

Keywords: parasite, host, population, relationships, physiology, biochemistry, histostructure, *Schistosoma turkestanicum*

1. Introduction

Trematodes *Sch. turkestanicum* are common for the biogeocenoses of the Indo-Malesian and Palaearctic, forming a part of the tropic and subtropic fauna. They have developed the ability to parasitise the blood vessels of mammals. Some populations were recorded in the Asian and European biogeocenoses; they cause serious diseases in animals and, therefore, great damage to the agriculture.

A population is a group of specimens of a certain species inhabiting a certain territory. Both free-living specimens of this territory and those living within the body of a host are considered to belong to the population inhabiting the territory [1].

As we noted before, apart from the parasite itself, the intermediate and definitive hosts participate in schistosoma's life cycle. Therefore, the structure of the population of this trematode is formed of groups characterised by the population's specific features (number, birth rate, death rate, sexes ratio, special distribution and so on) typical of the species.

Populations of the studied trematode include five interconnected groups of alternating parasitising and free-living states of a uniform process within the "parasite-host" system. The number of the free-living components is regulated by exogenous factors, and that of parasitising ones—by endogenous factors; that is, through the relations between a population of parasites with populations of corresponding hosts (**Table 1**).

As we have already noted, the following 17 mammal species were determined as definitive hosts in *Schistosoma turkestanicum* habitat: sheep, goat, cattle, buffalo, zebu, Arabian and Bactrian camels, saiga antelope, elk, deer, roe deer, horse, donkey, mule, wild boar, cat and rat. The intermediate hosts are four freshwater molluscs from the genus *Lymnaea*. Individual populations are associated with certain isolated territories within the habitats, where outbreaks of infection were recorded.

The infection circulates between the molluscs and mammals within some isolated territories of the habitat. The participation of some wild mammals (buffalo, zebu, saiga antelope, elk, deer, roe deer, wild boar and rat) in the circulation means the territory of natural outbreaks of *Sch. turkestanicum* is stable.

Trematode populations are not distributed evenly within the habitat, which is, probably, connected with the diverse conditions in different biospheric areas. The environmental conditions that met the life requirements of this species led to the concentration of this trematode in certain areas. The successful establishment of the "parasite-host" relations in these areas is determined the species' actual habitat. The degree of the isolation of this or that population is, apparently, connected with different levels of the mobility of *Sch. turkestanicum* hosts and with various barriers preventing the animals' migration. We suppose that initially these schistosomas used wild ungulates (buffalo, zebu, elk, deer, roe deer and saiga) as their definitive hosts; the second stage of distribution was the adaptation to domestic ungulates (horse, donkey, mule, sheep, goat, cattle and camel); and the third stage was characterised by increase of the range of hosts (rat, wild boar).

The stages we have just mentioned are doubtlessly associated with the distribution of the molluscs, the trematode's intermediate hosts.

The populations of maritae (mature trematodes) living in the blood vessels of mammals are divided into males and females. The males are usually more numerous. These trematodes reproduce themselves in the organism of the definitive host. The size of a population ranges greatly and depends on the species of the definitive host and its age and on the season. The largest populations occur in late summer and in

Populations	**State**	**Habitat (location)**
Maritae	Parasitising	Mammals' blood vessels
Eggs	Free-living	External environment
Miracidia	Free-living	Water
Sporocysts	Parasitising	Inner organs of aquatic molluscs
Cercariae	Free-living	Water
Schistosomula	Parasitising	Mammals' blood vessels

Table 1.
The structure of populations of Schistosoma turkestanicum Skrjabin, 1913.

autumn. Populations of infected hosts may contain hundreds of thousands of trematode specimens. Parthenogenetic generations and cercariae develop in the organisms of molluscs. The cercariae's emission is cyclic and depends on the living organisms' general biorhythms. According to observations carried out for many years, a cercaria population coming out of one mollusc within 24 hours may range between 3755 and 10,000 specimens [2].

Thus, the population of the trematode under study consists of free-living (eggs, miracidia and cercariae) and parasitic (parthenitae, schistosomula and maritae) forms.

This structure functions properly within the "parasite-host" system. The dynamism of the system (including all its components) depends on a complex of exogenous and endogenous factors. The increase of the free-living populations of this system is restricted by abiotic environmental factors. Therefore, the parasite is usually affected by the unfavourable environmental factors of the first and second category within the "parasite-host" relations. Trematodes have developed a number of adaptive and compensatory mechanisms (high fertility, parthenogenesis, taxes, life cycles synchronisation and others) to maintain the size of a population at a level best for the maintenance of species. These mechanisms ensure the balance between the populations of the parasite and the host.

The human's activity leading to numerous successions in biogeocenoses changes greatly the size of populations and their compositions and breaks the relations between organisms. The great changes in the living conditions of animal and plant communities connected with the human activity led to imbalance in the biogeocenosis. Some members of the communities find the new living conditions unfavourable and their numbers fall abruptly, while others even become extinct. On the other hand, for some species these new conditions prove favourable and their populations grow. For example, the large-scale amelioration and irrigation and the creation and use of a number of artificial reservoirs led to the increase of cercariae populations. As a result, heavy outbreaks of infection were recorded among animals and the populations of parasites within the cattle populations increased beyond the threshold in these territories, which led to enzootic infections and deaths of domestic animals at the farms of the Republic of Karakalpakstan and Khorezm Province.

It should be noted that the parasites accumulate in the organisms of infected hosts, which enlarges the habitats of the parasites and leads to infections in sensitive animals [2, 3]. In the wild, such situation is regulated by negative feedback in the "parasite-host" system. When anthropogenic factors influence biogeocenoses and create favourable conditions for an overpopulation of a parasite at all its ontogenetic stages, the mechanisms regulating the size of the population fail to function in time and the infected animals die. Correction of infection may help relieve the parasitic press.

Taking into account what we have mentioned above, we propose a differentiated approach to the study of parasites' role in the dynamics of communities—the natural and artificial ecosystems.

Physiological and biochemical aspects of the "parasite-host" relations are mentioned in case of infection with *Schistosoma turkestanicum*. The leaving of mature in blood, the laying of eggs and leaving of metabolic and decay products in the host's organs and the migration of the eggs inside the host's tissues—all these are factors determining the high pathogenicity of these trematodes for productive animals.

In this section, we shall attempt to show the regular malfunctions *Schistosoma* cause to the animals' organisms.

The paper electrophoresis method is used most commonly to examine proteins and protein fractions in blood serum in case of parasitic diseases. The electrophoretic analysis of blood serum proteins is also widely used in the veterinary science to diagnose diseases in animals, as the parasites causing diseases alter the amounts of proteins and the protein fractions ratio in the blood serum.

It was the first time that the electrophoretic method was used to study schistosomiasis in animals [4–6].

Changes in the serum proteins compositions are recorded in sheep infected with cercariae of *Schistosoma turkestanicum*, the changes occurring on the third day after the infection and continuing for the whole period of the disease.

Blood serum protein fractions change during the entire period of infection. Almost all of the experimental animals infected with different numbers of larvae showed the same character of changes in the blood proteins. The most noticeable changes were recorded in the proteins of sheep infected by large numbers of *Sch. turkestanicum* larvae.

The dynamics of the protein fractions changes in the experimental animals can be divided into three phases.

The first phase covers the period between the beginning of the infection and the 10th–15th day and is characterised by the decrease of the number of albumins, the minimal level of which is 44.2 ± 0.334–44.7 ± 1.036%. The decrease in the number of albumins in the blood of the sheep infected with *Sch. turkestanicum* is confirmed by the statistics. Thus, the amount of albumin in the reference animals was 50.8 ± 0.35 in the first phase of infection and that in the infected animals was equal to 44.2 ± 0.334% and 44.7 ± 1.036%, with a high degree of validity in the difference between the reference and experimental animals.

Globulin fractions were recorded to increase in amount in this phase, with an alpha globulin content ranging between 17.2 ± 0.453% and 21.3 ± 0.672%. The increase in the amount of alpha globulin in the blood serum of the sheep infected with schistosoma in this phase is confirmed statistically. Thus, before infection the amount of alpha globulin in the sheep's blood serum was 12.0 ± 0.328% and 15.0 ± 0.025%, and three days after infection, it was equal to 21.3 + 0.672%, the validity of data being confirmed by both the pre-infection figures and the reference animals (td = 6.7). The variation of beta globulin was not considerable—between 10.8 + 1.816% and 15.6 ± 0.794%. This variation was invalid (td = 1.4). Gamma globulin was constantly increasing in animals infected with 5000 cercariae. In this case, the ratio was 21.2 ± 0.52% to 26.0 ± 0.564%. The amount of gamma globulin was decreasing in sheep infected with 3000 cercariae—15.1 ± 1.773% and 11.3 ± 0.558%.

The first phase of the changes in the blood serum protein fractions coincided with the first stage of the clinical presentations of the disease in the experimental animals.

The degree of the deviation of the clinical and physiological values from the norm and the changes in the biochemistry of blood are associated with the penetration of the cercariae into the skin of the animal and the migration of young and developing schistosomules within the tissues and organs of the animal, damaging these organs, which causes the disease called cercarioses.

In our opinion, the changes in the blood serum protein fractions are the response of the macro-organism to the extreme activity of the larvae and their metabolites, which is accompanied by the physiological malfunction of haemopoietic organs.

In the second phase, which lasted from the 10th–13th day after the infection to the 40th day, the changes of the blood serum proteins compositions were not so obvious. However, the amount of albumin lowered from 41.4 ± 1.184% to 33.8 ± 1.777%.

The amount of alpha globulin also decreased somewhat. Its content in the blood serum was 14.5 ± 3.200%, which was almost within the norm. Certainly, the degree of the difference between the amounts of alpha globulin in the reference and experimental animals was not valid in this phase of infection. The amount of beta globulin, however, increased in the animals infected with large numbers of cercariae. On the 40th day after infection the beta globulin content was 17.6 ± 3.276%.The content of this component in the blood of the animals infected with small numbers of cercariae remained within the norm or decreased slightly—13.1 ± 0.040% and 11.8 ± 1.411%. The amount of gamma globulin in the animals infected with large numbers of schistosoma cercariae (5000) continued to increase constantly. The gamma globulin content was 26.0 ± 0.564%. The amount of gamma globulin in the blood serum of the animals infected with small numbers (3000) of larvae lowered to 11.8 ± 0.558% by the 20th day, while the content of this fraction in the reference animals was 15.1 ± 1.773%.

Therefore, the second phase of the blood serum protein changes in sheep has the following characteristics: considerable decrease in the amount of albumin, slight decrease in the amounts of beta and gamma globulins and the increase in the amount of alpha globulin.

Thus, the second phase of the blood serum protein changes coincides with the second stage of the disease, at which no obvious clinical presentations of schistosomiasis are recorded.

However, it is obvious that at this stage of infection quantitative and qualitative changes in the blood protein fractions occur, characterised by the decrease in the amounts of albumin and beta and gamma globulin and the increase in the amounts of alpha globulin.

The third phase of the changes in the blood protein formula covers the period from the 40th day to the end of the experiment and is characterised by a spasmodic increase in the amount of gamma globulin. The gamma globulin fraction content on the 40th day after the infection was 20.8 ± 0.4215% and 27.3 ± 1.436%. On the 70th day after infection the gamma globulin ratio in the blood serum was 28.0 ± 1.294 to 34.4 ± 1.978%, with a high degree of validity (td = 9.3). In the same period, beta globulin ranged between 17.6 ± 0.277 and 20.5 ± 0.29%. The increase in the amount of beta globulin in the blood of animals infected with schistosoma cercariae is confirmed statistically. So, in three months the amount of beta globulin in the reference animals was equal to 14.0 ± 0.286%, and in the experimental animals—up to 0.5 ± 0.299% in the same period. Therefore, the increase of this component in the blood serum of the sheep infected with schistosoma is statistically valid (td = 15.8).

The amount of alpha globulin in the animals infected with relatively small numbers of cercariae ranged between 14.5 ± 0.200% and 15.9 ± 0.61% in this phase. The other group of sheep, infected with large numbers of larvae, demonstrated slight increase in the amount of alpha globulin—16.3 ± 0.276% and 17.7 ± 0.327%. However, these changes proved to be invalid (td = 0.5).

Since the 40th day of infection the amount of albumin decreased rapidly to 38.8 ± 1.777% and reaches a minimum of 29.0 ± 1.425% in 70 days. The decrease in the amount of albumin in the blood of the sheep infected with schistosoma is statistically valid. So the average arithmetical values of the albumin in the blood serum of the reference animals were equal to 50.2 ± 0.577%, in the third phase of the infection, while that in the experimental animals was 29.0 ± 1.425%, with a high degree of validity comparing with the test data (td = 13.3). Further the albumin content increases slightly, approaching the norm; however, it never reaches the norm, even 100 days after the infection (41.5 ± 1.291%).

Therefore, the change of the blood serum protein fractions in case of schistosomiasis in this phase coincides with the third stage of the disease, which is characterised by the parasitising with mature trematode specimens, the laying of eggs in the vessels and the migration of the eggs within the organs and tissues of the animal.

In the course of the research, we established that the dynamics of the changes of the blood protein fractions remains qualitatively the same in the animals infected with different numbers of larvae. However, the changes in the proteins are more obvious in the animals infected by large numbers of cercariae.

Thus, this infection leads to considerable clinical, physiological and functional changes in the organisms of animals; in particular, it changes the blood protein fractions ratio. The changes reflect the considerable physiological and immunological restructuring of the organism.

We established that cercariae of trematodes cause morphological changes and physical and chemical in the blood of the infected sheep.

In the first phase of the disease haemoglobin rises slightly—13.0 ± 0.654% and 13.9 ± 0.434%, which is statistically invalid.

In 3 to 10 days after infection the number of erythrocytes increases to 13.7 ± 0.877% and 14.0 ± 0.032, which is statistically valid (td = 11.4). The same valid differences were recorded between the increase of leukocytes in the reference and experimental animals. We also recorded considerable increase in the quantity of eosinophils in the blood—4.8 ± 1.145% and 5.8 ± 1.099%. The validity of the changes of this blood component in the reference and experimental animals at this stage of the disease is doubtless.

The data we obtained testify to a decrease of the blood alkali reserve in the sheep in the first phase of the infection. In 10 days after infection the alkali reserve of the experimental animals was equal to 442 ± 33.374% and 458 ± 1.367%, while that of the reference animals—458 ± 1.367 and 490 ± 8.328%. The difference in this blood component between the experimental and reference animals is obvious (td = 3.4).

We recorded slight decrease in the amount of sugar in the blood 3 to 10 days after infection of the sheep with schistosoma. However, this decrease was not statistically valid (td = 1.9).

The second phase of the disease lasts for 5–6 weeks. Haemoglobin ranges between 10.8 ± 0.251 and 12.4 ± 0.263 mg%.

The number of erythrocytes and leukocytes remains within the physiological norm. However, the amount of eosinophil increased noticeably—4.0 ± 0.282 and 5.0 ± 0.721 mg%. The increase in the amount of eosinophil in this phase of the disease was statistically valid (td = 4.9). We recorded slight changes in the physical and chemical composition of the blood in the experimental animals.

The third phase of the disease begins in 5–6 weeks after the animal was infected and is characterised by great changes in the haemopoietic organs and metabolic processes. When the disease developed, we recorded decrease in the amount of haemoglobin—6.06 ± 1.101% and 8.2 ± 0.908 mg%, which is statistically valid (td = 5.05).

We recorded some decrease in the quantity of erythrocytes—to 7.7 ± 0.687 million and increase in the number of leukocytes—to 14.2 ± 1.084 thousand. These changes in the experimental animals proved to be statistically valid in this phase of disease—td = 3.5 and 7.6, respectively (**Figure 1**).

The increase in the number of eosinophils in the blood was the most noticeable. In 40–50 days after infection their quantity increased spasmodically to 25.0 ± 5.831 and 33.0 ± 5.062, which is highly valid (td = 6.1). No obvious changes were recorded in the quantity of leukocytes.

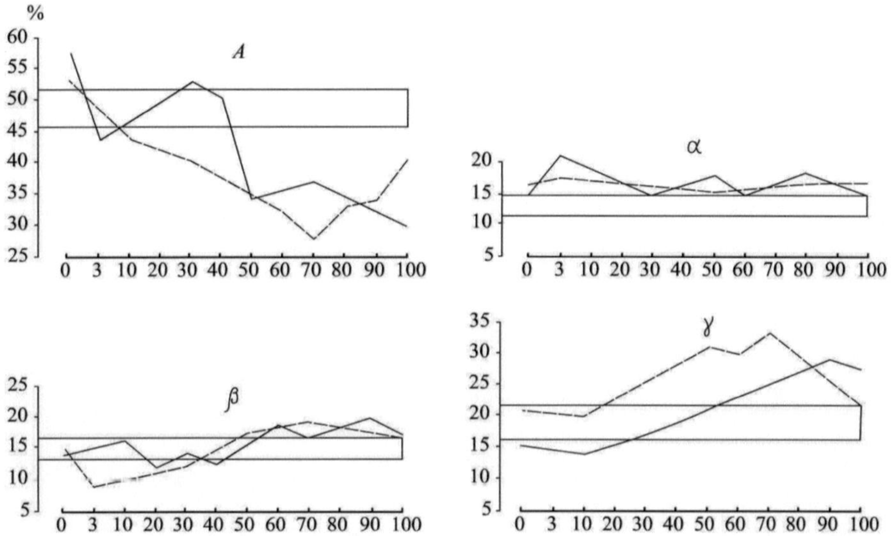

Figure 1.
The dynamics of changes in the amounts of protein fractions in the blood serum of sheep after they were infected with schistosoma cercariae: Continuous line—Sheep infected with 3000 cercariae; dashed line—Sheep infected with 5000 cercariae; A—Albumin, α-, β-, γ-globulin [7].

The alkali reserve of the blood serum in the experimental animals was equal to 457 ± 0.658 and 524 ± 13.144 mg% prior to their infection with *Schistosoma* cercariae. In the acute phase of the disease, the blood alkali reserve decreased to 336 ± 8.944 mg%, while in the reference animals it was 457 ± 0.658 mg%. The decrease of the alkali reserve in the blood of the experimental animals in comparison with the reference animals proved to be highly valid (td = 13.5).

As we know, the buffer imbalance in the organism leads to the malfunction of enzymatic processes in the tissues, which impacts greatly the principal metabolic processes, including the carbohydrate metabolism.

We recorded decrease in the sugar content in the blood in 40–50 days after the animals were infected with *Schistosoma* to 82.0 ± 3.364 and 87.6 ± 6.748 mg %. Then, we recorded an abrupt decrease of this blood component to 45.0 ± 2.508 mg %. The decrease of sugar content in the blood of sheep is statistically valid. Thus, the sugar content in the blood of the reference animals ranged within the physiological norm (between 90.0 ± 0.282 and 106.0 ± 1.190 mg %) throughout the experiment, while the experimental animals did not demonstrate this stability. The sugar content in their blood tends to lower, with a minimum recorded at the acute stage of the disease—45.0 ± 2.508 and 74.0 ± 2.190 mg % with a high statistical validity (td = 21.9).

Thus, the acute phase of the disease is characterised by clinical and morphological changes in the organisms of the animals. *Schistosoma* blocks the vessels, which leads to oedema. The metabolic and blood formation processes also function improperly and the physical and chemical properties of blood change, which is confirmed by the research carried out by Zakhryalov (1975).

Transition into the chronic form. This phase is characterised by changes similar to those in the third phase of the disease, which, however, are not so obvious; this is conditioned by tissular proliferation and gradual restoration of the tissues' function (**Figure 2**).

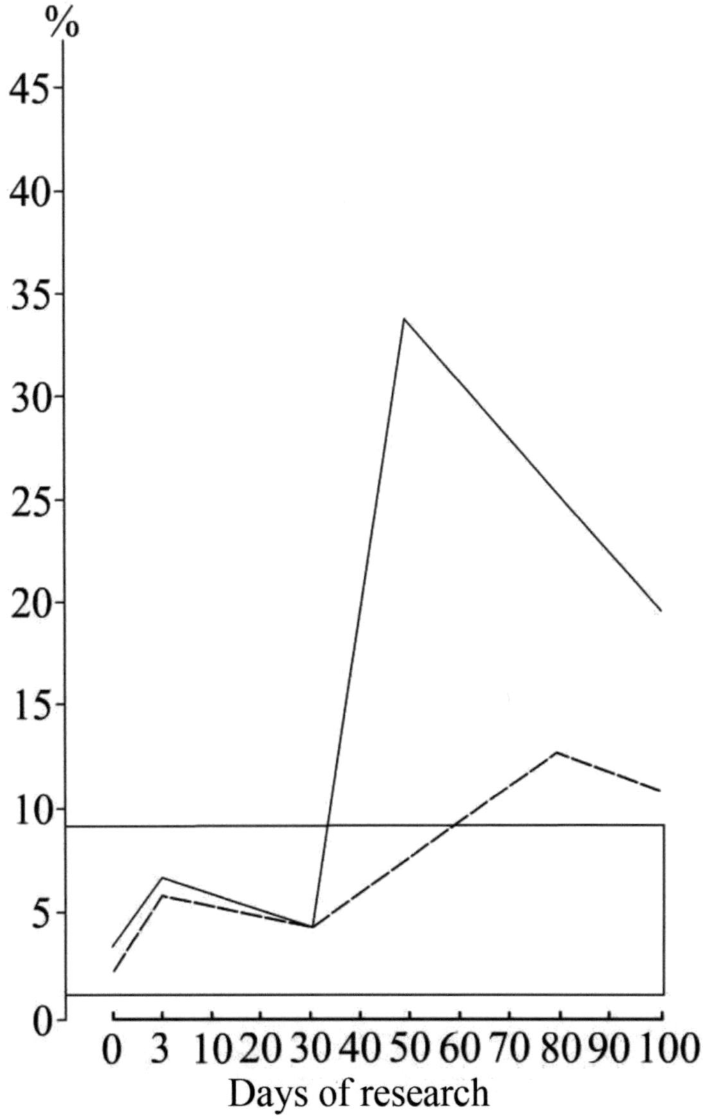

Figure 2.
The dynamics of changes in the amounts of eosinophil in the blood of sheep infected with Schistosoma turkestanicum (A) and the dynamics of changes in the amounts of sugar in the blood of sheep infected with Schistosoma turkestanicum *(B) - - - - sheep infected by 3000 cercariae, sheep infected by 5000 cercariae [7].*

The trematode's pathogenic influence on the organisms of the animals' results from the mechanic destruction of the host's tissues by the cercariae as they penetrate into it and migrate within it (cercariosis); the mechanic destruction by mature trematodes (thrombosis and rupture of blood vessels); the traumatism of the organs and tissues by the migrating eggs; the intoxication of the hosts organs and tissues by metabolic and decay products; the allergic response [3, 5].

Phospholipid and fatty acid compositions of the tissues of trematode *Schistosoma turkestanicum*. To study the biochemical aspects of the relations of *Sch. turkestanicum* within the "parasite-host" relations, we researched into the phospholipids and their fatty acids in mature trematodes, the content of phospholipid fractions and fatty acids in the liver of molluscs *Lymnaea auricularia*, *Sch. turkestanicum* intermediate hosts and the influence of the parasite on the content of the abovementioned components in definitive hosts.

We should note that the "parasite-host" system forms at the moment when the miracidia penetrate into the molluscs' organisms (the first stage of the development of the system) and the cercariae into the organisms of vertebrates (the second stage).

The concentration of helminths in different tissues of their host must affect the chemical composition of the parasites' tissue, in particular, phospholipids and fatty acids.

The comparative study of the phospholipid composition of *Sch. turkestanicum* and *Fasciola gigantica* demonstrates that the qualitative composition of the phospholipid fractions is the same, but their quantities are different (**Table 2**).

Phosphatidylcholine and phosphatidylethanolamine were the most massive phospholipid fractions. Phosphatidylcholine is the main phospholipid component in whole organ and tissues, as well as in various subcellular organelles in different animals, including helminths, and is a more saturated phospholipid than phosphatidylethanolamine [8].

The roles it plays in the cell are diverse; however, its main function is that it is a "structural phospholipid" and, together with phosphatidylethanolamine, is an essential component in many enzymatic systems. Phosphatidylcholine is the most labile and highly metabolic phospholipid, which performs both the reserve and the energising function in the cell [9]. In addition, phosphatidylcholine is a structural component in the cell membrane of animals with low lipid content and performs the same function as the reserve lipid triacetilglicerin [10].

Phosphatidylethanolamine, like other phospholipids, react specific environmental conditions, temperature and pressure, changing its fatty acid composition [11] and is the most saturated of the phospholipids.

It should be noted that the total amount of phosphatidylcholine and phosphatidylethanolamine is 70.1% (here and further in the text: of the total amount of phospholipids) in both helminths. However, the two chemicals are present in different

No.	Phospholipid fractions	*Sch. turkestanicum* (n = 100)	*F. gigantica* (n = 12)
1	Phosphatidylcholine	38.8 ± 1.5	46.6 ± 1.3
2	Phosphatidylethanolamine	31.3 ± 1.8	23.5 ± 0.8
3	Cardiolipin	4.7 ± 0.5	6.5 ± 0.5
4	Phosphatidic acid	5.7 ± 0.7	1.1 ± 0.2
5	Sphingomyelin	6.1 ± 0.6	4.5 ± 0.4
6	Phosphatidyl serine	7.9 ± 0.3	12.3 ± 0.7
7	Phosphatidyl inositol	Traces	Traces
8	Lysophosphatidylcholine	3.0 ± 0.2	3.2 ± 0.3
9	Lysophosphatidylethanolamine	0.9 ± 0.1	1.3 ± 0.2
10	Unidentified phospholipids	1.6 ± 0.2	1.4 ± 0.1

Note: confidence intervals were calculated at a probability level of 0.01.

Table 2.
The content of phospholipid fractions in the homogenate of Sch. turkestanicum and Fasciola gigantica (M ± m) (phospholipids in per cent of the amount of all phospholipids).

proportions. So the phosphatidylcholine content in the tissue of *Sch. turkestanicum* is less than 38.8%, while that of *Fasciola gigantica* is 46.6%; on the other hand, *Sch. turkestanicum* contains more phosphatidylethanolamine (31.3%, with 23.5% in *F. gigantica*).

We noted that *Sch. turkestanicum* contains more phosphatidic acid (5.7%) than *F. gigantica* does (1.1%). The cell membrane contains small amounts of phosphatidic acid; however, it is an important intermediate product of the biosynthesis of other phospholipids. In addition, phosphatidic acid performs an ionophore function, participating in the formation of ion channels [11].

Phosphatidyl serine is the third phospholipid in the homogenates of both species by its relative content. The amount of phosphatidyl serine in *Sch. turkestanicum* is 1.5 smaller than that in *F. gigantica*. Phosphatidyl serine in invertebrates, by analogy with fish and mammals, may participate in the formation of eicosanoids and leukotrienes, regulate the transportation of ions through the membranes and speed up metabolism [10].

Both helminth species contain high amounts of cardiolipin comparing either invertebrates. As we know, cardiolipin is the most specific phospholipid to the mitochondrial membrane [11–13] and this phospholipid is one of the components of the respiratory enzymes of the mitochondria, where it helps stimulate the transfer of ions on the membrane [9].

Does it mean trematodes contain high concentrations of mitochondria?

One of the signs of a living organism's evolutionary level is the sphingomyelin content. Both helminths contain rather small amounts of sphingomyelin.

The two helminth species differ considerably in the quantitative content of certain phospholipid fractions in their tissues, which may be connected with the taxonomic diversity and the parasites' adaptation to different habitats (their hosts having different tissues).

The difference in the phospholipid composition encouraged us to examine the fatty acid composition of total phospholipids. The gas-liquid chromatography we used to analyse the methyl ethers of the fatty acids of general phospholipids allowed us to identify 9 fractions in *Sch. turkestanicum* and 10 fractions in *F. gigantica* (**Table 3**).

Ectothermic organisms react changes in the environment, which can break the normal structure and functioning of biological membranes by making changes in the properties of the lipids included in the membranes. These changes relate, first of all, the fatty acid composition of the membranes' phospholipids.As we can see in **Table 3**, unsaturated fatty acids predominate over saturated ones. Both in *Sch. turkestanicum* and in *Fasciola gigantica* saturated fatty acids comprise myristinic and stearic acids, while the unsaturated ones consist of oleic and arachidonic acids. The total amount of saturated fatty acids in the tissues of *Sch. turkestanicum* is 44.5%, and 39.7% in *F. gigantica*, while the total amount of oleic and arachidonic acids in the first species is 43.0% of the amount of all fatty acids or 77.5% of the quantity of all unsaturated fatty acids, while in the second species the amount is only 32.0% or 60.0% of the quantity of all unsaturated fatty acids. The palmitoleic acid content in *F. gigantica* is 3.2 times higher than in the other species. The ratio of unsaturated fatty acids to saturated fatty acids is 1.25:1 in *Schistosoma* and 1.34:1 in *Fasciola*.

The results of the research allow us to conclude the qualitative and quantitative content of fatty acid phospholipid fractions in the tissues of the helminths depends on the place the parasite occupies in the organ.

No.	Fatty acids	*Sch. turkestanicum* (n = 100)	*F. gigantica* (n = 12)
1	Lauric (12:0)	2.1 ± 0.2	0.6 ± 0.06
2	Myristoleic (14:1)	2.2 ± 0.1	1.3 ± 0.1
3	Myristinic (14:0)	20.0 ± 1.1	25.6 ± 0.5
4	Palmitoleic (16:1)	3.8 ± 0.3	12.3 ± 1.0
5	Palmitic (16:0)	3.4 ± 0.4	3.3 ± 0.2
6	Linoleic (18:2)	—	2.8 ± 0.3
7	Oleic (18:1)	26.5 ± 1.9	19.6 ± 1.4
8	Stearic (18:0)	18.1 ± 1.4	10.2 ± 0.8
9	Arachidonic (20:4)	18.5 ± 1.2	12.4 ± 0.4
10	Docosatetraenoic (22:4)	8.5 ± 0.5	4.6 ± 0.4
11	Unidentified fatty acids	—	6.5 ± 0.5
12	Saturated	44.5%	39.7%
13	Unsaturated	55.5%	53.2
14	Unsaturated Saturated	1.25	1.34

Note: the first number after the name of the acid is the number of carbon atoms in the hydrocarbon chain, the second one—the number of double bonds. The confidence intervals were calculated at a probability level of 0.01.

Table 3.
The fatty acid composition of the total phospholipids of Sch. turkestanicum and Fasciola gigantica (M ± m) (in % of the number of fatty acids).

Thus, in the course of the evolution of the "parasite-host" system the helminths developed a mechanism forming a composition of phospholipids and their component fatty acid fractions, where they are present in proportions necessary for the parasites' vital functions [2, 14, 15]. Other scientists have similar viewpoints on vertebrate animals [11, 13].

The content of phospholipid and fatty-acid fractions in the liver of molluscs *Lymnaea auricularia*. The parthenogenetic trematode generations parasitising molluscs have a negative impact of the vital functions of the host. This impact shows itself in the parasitic castration of the molluscs, the decrease of the reserve nutrients content and haemoglobin in the haemolymph in infected specimens [16], the increase of the heart rate and so on.

Helminths are supposed to affect the structural and functional characteristics of the host's cell membranes [8]. In the first place, this is reflected by the composition of phospholipids participating in biological processes, in particular, in the organism's adaptation to the environment [11].

In this section, we plan to study the impact of parthenitae of trematode *Sch. turkestanicum* on the phospholipid status of the liver of freshwater molluscs *L. auricularia.*

The analysis showed that the total amount of phospholipids in the liver homogenate in uninfected molluscs is 40.0 mg/g of proteins, and 150.0 mg/g in infected ones, which exceeds the norm almost four times. At the same time, the quantity of general protein becomes 6.6 times smaller in infected molluscs (145 mg/g of tissues in uninfected molluscs and 21.8 mg/g in infected ones). Other animals were also recorded to contain less protein when infected [17–20]. The portion of phospholipids per mollusc liver tissue remains almost the same after the infection. These figures may indicate that the protein-lipid balance of the molluscs' liver breaks as they become infected with parthenitae of the studied trematode.

The results of the thin-layer chromatography used to carry out a comparative study of the phospholipid composition of the homogenate of the liver of uninfected molluscs *L. auricularia* and those infected with parthenitae of trematode *Sch. turkestanicum* are given in **Table 4** and **Figure 3**. Most of the phospholipids in the liver of uninfected molluscs are phosphatidylcholine, the portion of which may reach 47.1% and thus corresponds with data from many other researchers on other mollusc species [21–25]. In terms of quantity, the next phospholipid fraction is phosphatidyl serine. The portion of phosphatidylcholine and phosphatidyl serine taken together is 62.0%.

Another fraction that comprises a large portion in the phospholipid composition of livers in most of vertebrates and invertebrates is phosphatidylethanolamine, the volume of which varies between 16% and 30%, and even more in some cases [11]. Unlike in other animal species, the phospholipid composition of the liver of molluscs *L. auricularia* is characterised by the low percentage of phosphatidylethanolamine, which is, probably, a feature specific to the taxon (**Table 4**). The portion of other identified phospholipids—phosphatidylinositols, cardiolipin, sphingomyelin, phosphatidic acid and lysoforms of phosphatidylcholine and phosphatidylethanolamine taken together is 16.8%, which corresponds with data on other vertebrates [11, 23].

The portion of certain phospholipid fractions in the liver of infected molluscs changes: the cardiolipin content rose 1.8 times and the sphingomyelin content increased 1.7 times, comparing with uninfected specimens, while the phosphatidylcholine content decreased 1.7 times and the phosphatidyl serine content—1.9 times.

The portion of lysophosphatidylcholine, the product of phosphatidylcholine degradation, rose greatly, having become 12 times as large. The increase in the quantity of lysophosphatidylcholine and the decrease in the amount of phosphatidylcholine mean that phospholipase A_2 activates when the mollusc is infected. Phospholipase A_2 hydrolysing phospholipids into fatty acids and lysophospholipids is an important element of the cell, which regulates directly the functional state of the cells.

No.	Phospholipid fractions	Uninfected liver (n = 50)	Infected liver (n = 50)
1	Phosphatidylcholine	47.1 ± 2.2	28.5 ± 1.5
2	Phosphatidylethanolamine	7.7 ± 0.5	8.6 ± 1.3
3	Cardiolipin	2.6 ± 0.5	4.6 ± 0.7
4	Phosphatidic acid	2.3 ± 0.3	3.7 ± 0.8
5	Sphingomyelin	4.0 ± 0.4	6.9 ± 0.9
6	Phosphatidyl serine	14.9 ± 0.4	7.5 ± 1.5
7	Lysophosphatidylcholine	1.3 ± 0.03	15.7 ± 1.6
8	Lysophosphatidylethanolamine	3.1 ± 0.4	3.6 ± 1.0
9	Phosphatidyl inositol	3.5 ± 0.4	5.4 ± 1.3
10	Unidentified phospholipids	13.5 ± 0.7	15.5 ± 0.5

Note: confidence intervals were calculated at a probability level of 0.01.

Table 4.
The phospholipid fractions content in the homogenate of the liver of molluscs Lymnaea auricularia infected and not infected with parthenitae of Sch. Turkestanicum (M ± m) (in % of the amount of all phospholipids).

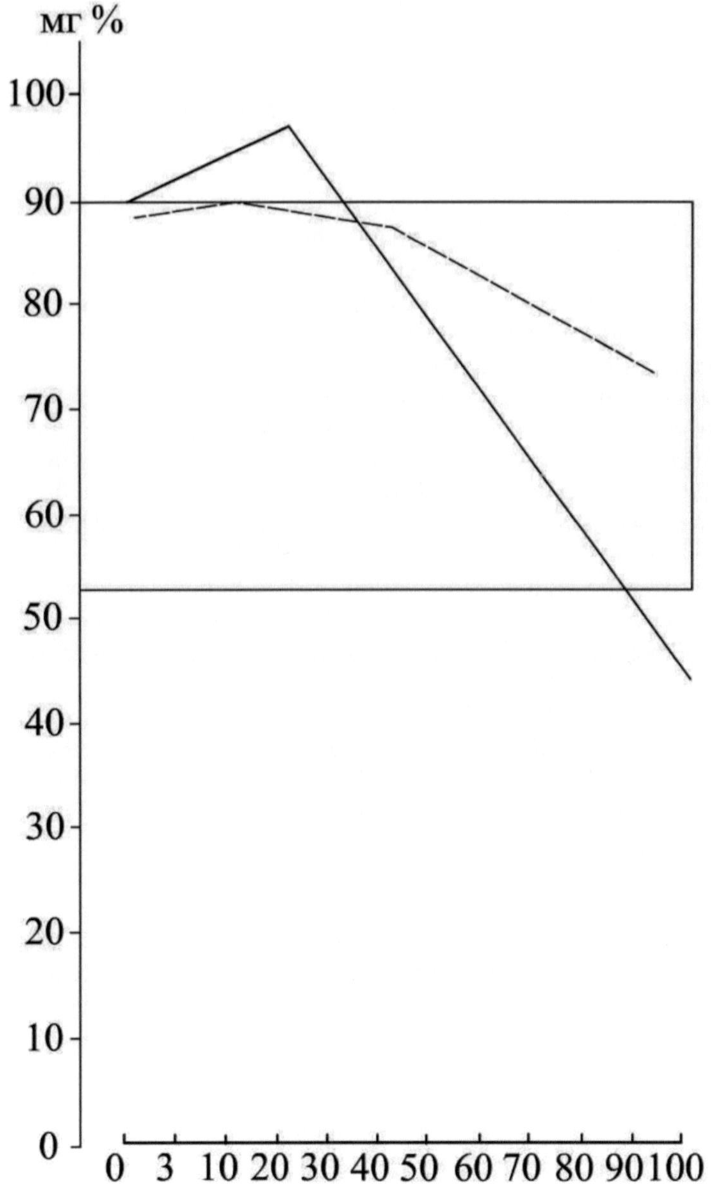

Figure 3.
The dynamics of changes in the amounts of sugar in the blood of sheep infected by Schistosoma turkestanicum (A) and the dynamics of changes in the amounts of sugar in the blood of sheep infected with Schistosoma turkestanicum. *(B) - - - - sheep infected by 3000 cercariae, sheep infected by 5000 cercariae.*

As we know, under normal conditions the endogenous phospholipases of the membranes are involved in the organism's adaptation to changing environment, while under stress or in pathologic situations they contribute to formation of "concealed" damaged membranes [26]. The high content of lysophosphatidylcholine among the phospholipids is one of the factors suppressing phosphorylation, inhibiting bound enzymes and breaking the membranes' structure. The increase in the amount of lysophospholipids means that the membranes' structures undergo changes that may lead to a necrosis of tissues, as lysophosphatidylcholine has detergent and haemolysing properties [27, 28].

In addition, the increase of the quantity of cardiolipin may be conditioned by the change in the activity of the tissue respiration enzymes under pathologic conditions [29].

Thus, we suppose that parthenitae of trematode *Sch. turkestanicum* changes the quantity of certain phospholipid fractions in the liver of molluscs *L. auricularia*, particularly in lysophosphatidylcholine. It may lead to changes in the lipid-protein relations and damage of the membranes' structure. Such disorder in the phospholipid component of the biomembranes leads to decrease of their permeability, which is just what the parasite needs to function properly [13].

The reason why the portion of phosphatidylethanolamine is somewhat smaller in the liver of the mollusc *L. auricularia* remains unknown currently. Nevertheless, the phosphatidylethanolamine and lysophosphatidylcholine contents in the livers of molluscs infected with parthenitae *Sch. turkestanicum* and their ratio (**Table 5**) are a criterion that allows us to estimate, in which direction the phospholipid composition changes.

We know that the fatty acid composition of phospholipids is the most sensible to changes in the environment [11]. Therefore, the environmental conditions or various damaging factors lead, first of all, to modification of the fatty acids and phospholipids in the cell membranes [30].

The results of the gas-liquid chromatography, which was used to analyse the fatty acid composition of the phospholipids in the livers of the molluscs infected and not infected with the parthenitae are given in **Table 5** and **Figure 4**. See **Figure 5**.

We identified 12 fatty acid fractions of general phospholipids in the liver of *L. auricularia*.

The fatty acids of the phospholipids in the liver of uninfected molluscs consist mainly of long-chain polyunsaturated fatty acids, consisting of 20 and 22 carbon atoms, which comprise 54%, with the total amount of unsaturated fatty acids being equal to 85.6%. When the polyene fatty acid content is high, the diffusion of chemicals through the membrane may run 20 times as fast than through the membranes containing only saturated fatty acids [12]. Polyunsaturated are considered to form specific microenvironment in the biological membrane, which helps the enzymatic systems function properly. The change in the microviscosity of the membranes leads to increased or decreased metabolism in the integral protein enzymes [31].

Thus, comparative research into the phospholipid composition of the liver of infected and uninfected cattle showed that the infection with trematodes *Sch. turkestanicum* changes the structure of the membranes. The phospholipid fractions may transmute in the infected liver, which is reflected in the change of their ratios. This may be caused by the excess activity of phospholipases, which is confirmed by the increased quantities of phospholipid lysoforms. Phospholipase A_2 contributes to the separation of unsaturated fatty acids, in particular, arachidonic acid, from the phospholipids, mainly from phosphatidylcholine and phosphatidylethanolamine [32]. Fatty acids can make the cell membranes more permeable for ions and some water-soluble substances [33]. In addition, arachidonic acid is capable of transforming into active effectors, namely, prostaglandins, leukotrienes and thromboxanes through a series of reactions. The second element produced by the effect of phospholipase A_2 on phosphatidylcholine, in most cases, is a lysoform of phosphatidylcholine.

No.	Fatty acids	Uninfected molluscs (n = 50)	Infected molluscs (n = 50)
1	Lauric (12:0)	0.9 ± 0.05	1.1 ± 0.05
2	Myristoleic (14:1)	0.4 ± 0.07	2.0 ± 0.2
3	Myristinic (14:0)	5.6 ± 0.5	3.8 ± 0.3
4	Palmitoleic (16:1)	2.2 ± 0.03	4.5 ± 0.3
5	Palmitic (16:0)	1.5 ± 0.1	4.2 ± 0.2
6	Linoleic (18:2)	2.5 ± 0.3	2.7 ± 0.05
7	Oleic (18:1)	19.4 ± 1.5	24.9 ± 1.0
8	Stearic (18:0)	4.3 ± 0.2	6.6 ± 0.7
9	Nonadecanoic (19:1)	7.2 ± 0.4	3.1 ± 0.1
10	Arachidonic (20:4)	19.7 ± 0.5	11.2 ± 0.6
11	Docosahexaenoic (22:6)	19.0 ± 0.2	13.1 ± 0.1
12	Docosatetraenoic (22:4)	15.3 ± 1.2	16.8 ± 0.9
13	Unidentified fatty acids	2.1 ± 0.5	5.7 ± 0.9
14	Saturated	12.8 ± 0.8	15.7 ± 0.7
15	Unsaturated	85.6 ± 1.5	78.3 ± 1.3
16	Unsaturated Saturated	7.0	5.0

Note: the first number after the name of the acid is the number of carbon atoms in the carbon chain, the second one—the number of double bonds. Confidence intervals were calculated at a probability level of 0.01.

Table 5.
The fatty acid composition of general phospholipids in the homogenate of the liver of Lymnaea auricularia infected and not infected with parthenitae of Sch. turkestanicum (M ± m) (in % of the amount of all fatty acids).

The portion of saturated fatty acids in the phospholipids is 12.3%, most of which are short-chain fatty acids (from 12 to 16 carbon atoms in a chain).

The principal fatty acid fractions in the phospholipids of the liver of uninfected molluscs *Lymnaea auricularia* are oleic, arachidonic, docosatetraenoic and docosahexaenoic unsaturated fatty acids, the total portion of which is 85.7% of the whole quantity of unsaturated fatty acids.

The high degree of unsaturation of the fatty acids in the liver of freshwater molluscs may be conditioned by their lifestyle, in particular, food and temperature. It was established that the food of the members of the trophic chain of the freshwater fauna contains large amounts of polyene fatty acids [34]. Although the fatty acids in the food lipids may have some effect on the fatty acid composition of phospholipids in various organs of poikilothermal animals, the insignificant differences in the winter time (which was observed in fish feeding properly and that starving) [13], apparently, testifies to the endogenous origin of the long-chain unsaturated acids in the phospholipids.

The molluscs infected with *Sch. turkestanicum* parthenitae have a phospholipid fatty acid composition in the liver, which is qualitatively different from that uninfected molluscs have; however, changes in the quantity of some fractions of fatty acids, in particular, myristoleic, palmitoleic, palmitic, oleic, nonadecanoic, arachidonic and docosahexaenoic acids, can also be observed. Moreover, these changes

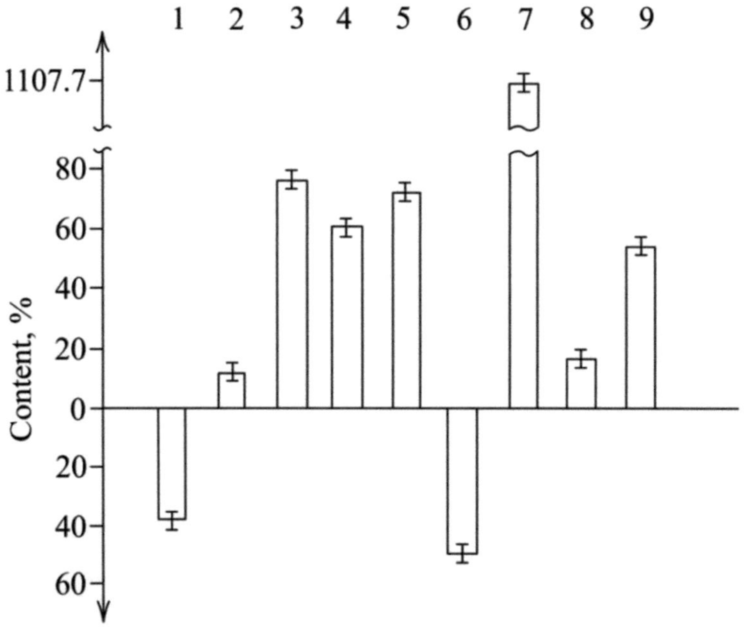

Figure 4.
Relative changes in the phospholipid composition of the liver homogenate in the liver of molluscs Lymnaea auricularia infected with parthenitae of Sch. turkestanicum: 1—Phosphatidylcholine; 2—Phosphatidylethanolamine; 3—Cardiolipin; 4—Phosphatidic acid; 5—Sphingomyelin; 6—Phosphatidyl serine; 7—Lysophosphatidylcholine; 8—Lysophosphatidylethanolamine; 9—Phosphatidyl inositol. The figures obtained from uninfected molluscs are taken as zero levels. Up—Increase of proportion, down—Decrease of proportion [7].

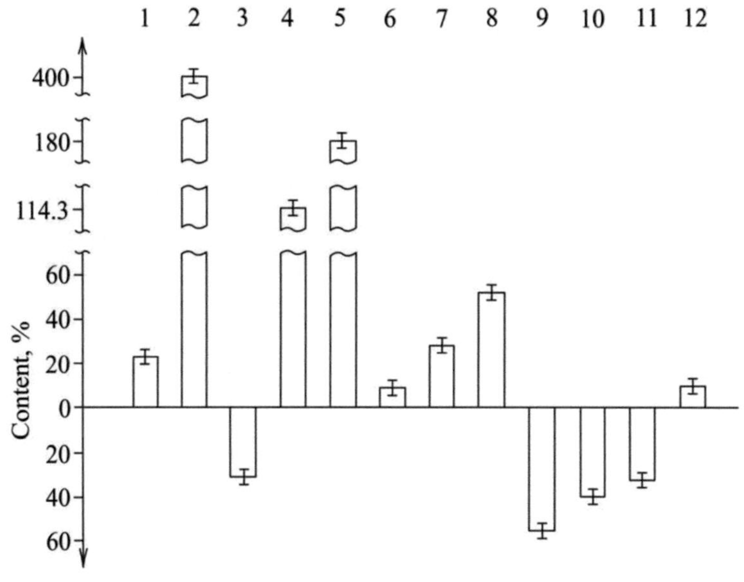

Figure 5.
The change in the fatty-acid composition of the general phospholipids in the homogenate of the liver of mollusc Lymnaea auricularia infected with parthenitae of Sch. turkestanicum. Acids: 1—Lauric; 2—Myristoleic; 3—Myristinic; 4—Palmitoleic; 5—Palmitic; 6—linoleic; 7—Oleic; 8—stearic; 9—Nonadecanoic; 10—arachidonic; 11—Docosahexaenoic; 12—Docosatetraenoic. The figures obtained from uninfected molluscs are taken as zero levels. Up—Increase of proportion, down—Decrease of proportion [7].

are interdependent. So, when the quantity of short-chain fatty acids increases, the amount of long-chain fatty acids decreases. In particular, the quantity of myristoleic acid increases 5 times, that of palmitoleic acid—2.1 times, palmitic acid—2.8 times and stearic acid—1.5 times. At the same time, the amounts of two massive fatty acids, arachidonic and docosahexaenoic, decrease 1.7 and 1.5 times, respectively, while the quantity of nonadecanoic acid becomes 2 times as small. We recorded that the content of the saturated fatty acids of the phospholipids in the livers of infected increased, while the amount of unsaturated fatty acids became smaller. Doubtless, the recorded changes in the composition of the phospholipid fatty acids and the phospholipids in the livers of infected molluscs reflect the structural changes in the cell membranes of the livers of molluscs infected with parthenitae of trematode *Sch. turkestanicum*.

The changes in the quantities of some phospholipid and fatty acid fractions in the livers of infected molluscs testify to changes in the barrier, transportation, structural and functional characteristics of the cell membranes, which, probably, reflects the enormity of pathologic changes in the whole organism.

The impact of schistosoma on the content of phospholipids and their fatty acids in the liver of cattle. The phospholipid composition of the liver of uninfected animals is characterised by high amounts of phosphatidylcholine and phosphatidylethanolamine and low quantities of lysophosphatidylcholine and lysophosphatidylethanolamine (**Table 6**). The total amount of phosphatidylcholine and phosphatidylethanolamine is 74.6%, while that of cardiolipin, phosphatidic acid, sphingomyelin, phosphatidyl serine and phosphatidyl inositol is only 19.0%. The ratio of amino compound phospholipids (phosphatidylethanolamine, phosphatidyl serine and lysophosphatidylethanolamine) to choline compound phospholipids (phosphatidylcholine, sphingomyelin and lysophosphatidylcholine) in the liver of uninfected cattle is 0.73:1. The given data conform with data on a number of warm-blooded animals [35].

Studying the phospholipid composition of cattle's liver infected with trematodes *Sch. turkestanicum*, we detected a statistically valid interdependent change in the quantities of certain phospholipid fractions. Thus, we detected decrease of the amount of the main phospholipids in the livers of infected animals—phosphatidylcholine by 19.8% and phosphatidylethanolamine by 25.8% in comparison with uninfected animals, while lysophosphatidylcholine grew by 232.3% and lysophosphatidylethanolamine by 178.9%. We also detected statistically valid increase in the amount of cardiolipin, sphingomyelin, phosphatidyl serine and phosphatidyl inositol by 76.2%, 41.7%, 41.2% and 23.7%, respectively (**Figure 6**). The ratio of amino compound phospholipids to choline compound phospholipids is 0.7:1 in the liver of infected cattle, which approaches the figure of uninfected animals.

Lysophosphatidylcholine, which appears among the phospholipids of the membranes in the infected liver, is one of the factors suppressing phosphorylation. According to some scientists, the inhibited activity of the membrane-bound enzymes activates guanylate cyclase; that is, it can act as the cyclic guanosine monophosphate (cGMP) signal inductor [32].

Such modifications of the membrane structures may cause changes in the conformational, physical and chemical properties of the membrane proteins—the enzymes. In its turn, this leads to changes in the interactions of lipids with proteins and proteins with proteins in the membranes of the cells of the liver infected with trematode *Sch. turkestanicum*.

Comparing the available data allows us to talk about the principal similarity in the change of the phospholipid status in cattle and molluscs infected with

No.	Phospholipid fractions	Uninfected liver (n = 10)	Infected liver (n = 12)
1	Phosphatidylcholine	44.8 ± 2.4	35.9 ± 2.1
2	Phosphatidylethanolamine	29.8 ± 1.7	22.1 ± 1.9
3	Cardiolipin	2.1 ± 0.2	3.7 ± 0.4
4	Phosphatidic acid	1.5 ± 0.3	0.9 ± 0.1
5	Sphingomyelin	4.8 ± 0.6	6.8 ± 0.4
6	Phosphatidyl serine	6.8 ± 0.3	9.6 ± 0.9
7	Phosphatidyl inositol	3.8 ± 0.5	4.7 ± 0.4
8	Lysophosphatidylcholine	3.1 ± 0.3	10.3 ± 0.4
9	Lysophosphatidylethanolamine	1.9 ± 0.2	5.3 ± 0.7
10	Unidentified phospholipids	1.4 ± 0.2	0.8 ± 0.02

Note: confidence intervals were calculated at a probability level of 0.01.

Table 6.
The phospholipid fractions content in the homogenate of the liver of cattle infected and not infected with maritae of Sch. turkestanicum (M ± m) (in % of the amount of all phospholipids).

trematodes *Sch. turkestanicum* and thus confirms the existence of a single mechanism of breaking the membranes' structure. The change in the phospholipid composition in the liver of the molluscs is accompanied by interdependent changes and, possibly, transmutations and turning of some phospholipid fractions into some other phospholipid fractions: in particular, the decrease of the portion of phosphatidylcholine from 47.1% to 28.5% and considerable increase of lysophosphatidylcholine to 15.7 (12 times), cardiolipin 1.8 times and sphingomyelin 1.7 times.

According to these data, both parthenitae and mature trematodes *Sch. turkestanicum* produce similar structural modifications of the membranes of the liver cells in freshwater molluscs and cattle. At the same time, the membranes' ability to increase the activity of endogenous phospholipases A_2 in infected animals is a specific feature indicating their functional activity. In this connection, we suppose that the infection of the liver of cattle with *Sch. turkestanicum* predetermine such composition of the membranes and such principles of their organisation that decrease considerably their function, increasing, in the first place, the permeability of ions and some metabolites and low-molecular carbohydrates.

We identified 14 fatty acid fractions of general phospholipids in the liver of cattle. The unsaturated fatty acids in uninfected cattle comprise mainly oleic and docosatetraenoic fatty acids, their total amount being 60.1% of the total quantity of unsaturated fatty acids. The total amount of saturated fatty acids in the liver of cattle is 37.5 ± 0.5%, while the total amount of myristinic and stearic acids is 64.3% of the total of all saturated fatty acids.

The quantities of some fatty acid fractions in the general phospholipids in the liver of cattle infected with trematodes *Sch. turkestanicum* changes noticeably (**Table** 7; see Figure x, Chapter x). Thus, the total amount of saturated fatty acids in the liver of cattle decreases 1.4 times. At the same time, the decrease of the whole amount of saturated fatty acids was characterised by simultaneous increase of the content of unsaturated fatty acids of phospholipids 1.2 times. According to some scientists, the decrease

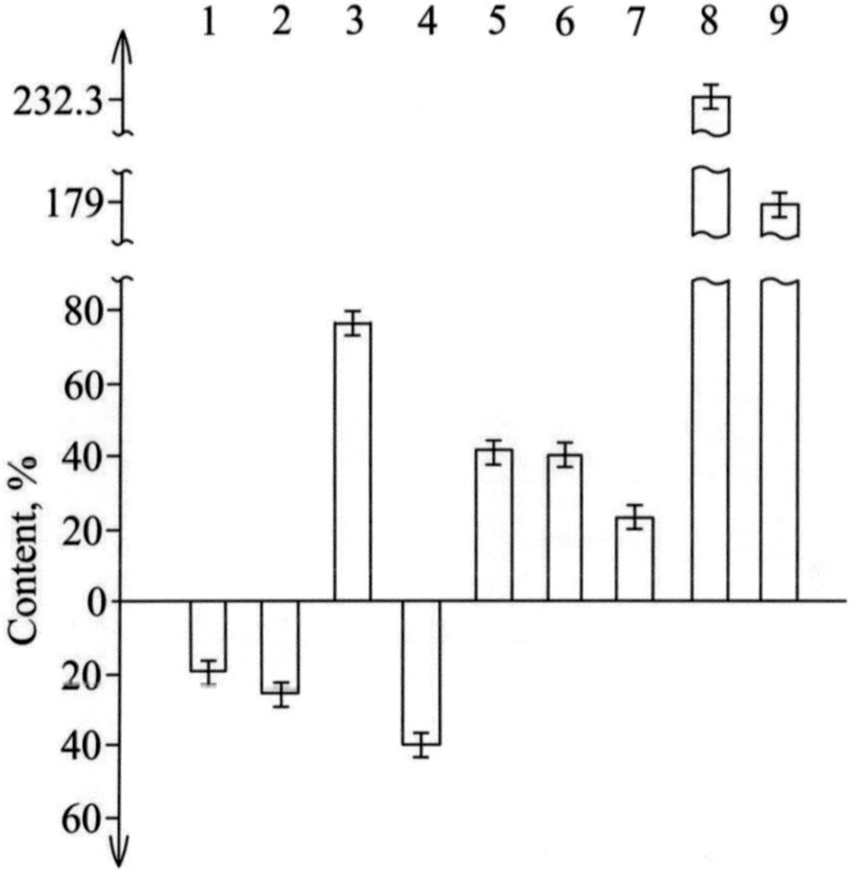

Figure 6.
Changes in the phospholipid composition of the liver homogenate in the liver of cattle infected with schistosoma: 1—Phosphatidylcholine; 2—Phosphatidylethanolamine; 3—Cardiolipin; 4—Phosphatidic acid; 5—Sphingomyelin; 6—Phosphatidyl serine; 7—Phosphatidyl inositol; 8—Lysophosphatidylcholine. The figures obtained from uninfected animals are taken as zero levels. Up—Increase of proportion, down—Decrease of proportion [7].

of the phospholipid hydrocarbon radical makes the membranes more permeable for ions and low-molecular metabolites [11, 13].

Some of the saturated fatty acids, in particular, lauric, myristinic, stearic and non-adecylic decrease by 68.4; 30.3; 28.8 and 55.8% respectively. The portion of palmitic acid increases by 63.2% (**Figure 7**). Palmitic acid is known to be the end product of the extramitochondrial enzymatic system of the biosynthesis of fatty acids in the liver and the source material for other endogenous higher fatty acids [36]. The increase in the portion of palmitic acid may be associated with the fatty acid synthesis becoming active [37].

Some of the unsaturated fatty acids, in particular, palmitoleic, linoleic, oleic and arachidonic acids, increase by 105.3; 20.9; 50.3 and 29.8% respectively, while docosa-tetraenoic acid decreases by 28.6%.

Thus, the results of the research given above demonstrated that the parasitising with maritae *Sch. turkestanicum* leads to changes in the lipidic metabolism in the liver of cattle.

No.	Fatty acids	Infected liver	Uninfected liver
1	Lauric (12:0)	1.9 ± 0.4	0.6 ± 0.1
2	Myristoleic (14:1)	2.3 ± 0.4	2.2 ± 0.1
3	Myristinic (14:0)	10.9 ± 0.1	7.6 ± 0.8
4	Hexadecadienoic (16:2)	0.6 ± 0.1	0.8 ± 0.1
5	Palmitoleic (16:1)	1.9 ± 0.1	3.9 ± 0.4
6	Palmitic (16:0)	3.8 ± 0.2	6.2 ± 0.6
7	Linoleic (18:2)	4.3 ± 0.5	5.2 ± 0.8
8	Oleic (18:1)	17.1 ± 0.6	25.7 ± 0.8
9	Stearic (18:0)	13.2 ± 0.7	9.4 ± .0.8
10	Nonadecanoic (19:1)	—	0.9 ± 0.1
11	Nonadecylic (19:0)	7.7 ± 0.1	3.4 ± 0.2
12	Arachidonic (20:4)	9.4 ± 0.7	12.2 ± 0.6
13	Docosahexaenoic (22:6)	5.6 ± 0.7	5.9 ± 0.2
14	Docosatetraenoic (22:4)	19.2 ± 0.5	13.7 ± 0.4
15	Unidentified fatty acids	2.1 ± 0.3	2.7 ± 0.2
Saturated		37.5 ± 0.5	27.2 ± 0.6
Unsaturated		60.4 ± 0.6	69.1 ± 0.8
Unsaturated Saturated		1.6	2.5

Note: confidence intervals were calculated at a probability level of 0.01.

Table 7.
The fatty acid composition of general phospholipids in the liver of cattle infected and not infected with schistosoma (M ± m) (in % of the amount of all fatty acids).

2. The changes in the histological structure of the hepatopancreas of molluscs *Lymnaea auricularia* (Linnaeus, 1758) parasitised with larvae of trematode *Schistosoma turkestanicum* Skrjabin, 1913

The parthenogenetic generations of trematodes parasitising the organism of the mollusc leads to malfunction in certain organs, often breaking the normal metabolism in the body of the host. The parthenitae's destructive effect may be conditioned by the mechanic destruction of the tissues of the host mollusc, taking of nutrients and the poisoning of the mollusc's organism with parthenitae metabolites [38].

In most cases, parthenitae concentrate in the mollusc's liver (hepatopancreas). It has secreting pancreatic cells scattered about it. This organ is a highly branchy tubular gland. The liver's main function is the intracellular digestion of proteins, fats and carbohydrates [38, 39]. The parasitising trematode larvae cause strong structural and functional changes in the liver and other organs of the mollusc [40–42]. Strong infection destroys the liver and may result in the molluscs' death [43].

According to a number of researchers [3, 44–48] parthenitae of Schistosomatidae and Bilharziellidae parasitise the molluscs' hepatopancreas alone. However, data on the changes in the structure of the molluscs' liver caused by parthenitae and cercariae of the mentioned trematodes are very fragmentary and insufficient. In this respect to

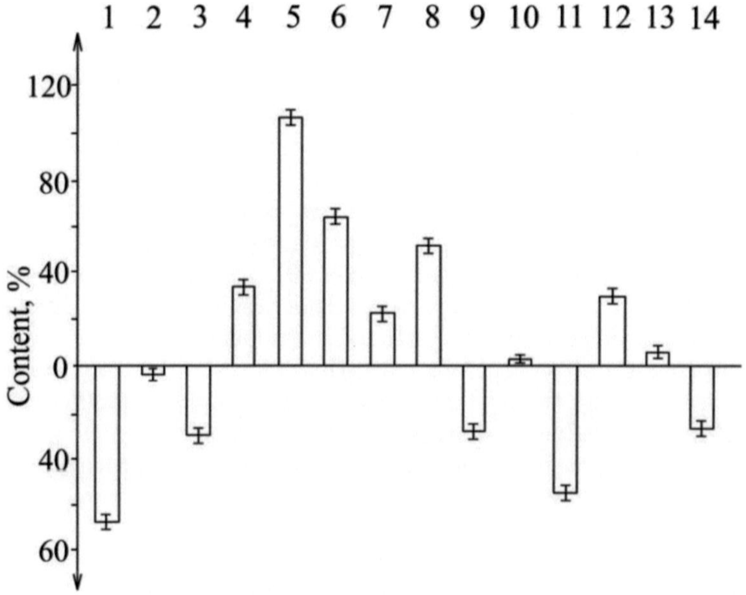

Figure 7.
The change in the fatty-acid composition of the general phospholipids in the homogenate of the liver of cattle infected with schistosoma. Acids: 1—Lauric; 2—Myristoleic; 3—Myristinic; 4—Hexadecadienoic; 5—Palmitoleic; 6—Palmitic; 7—Linoleic; 8—Oleic; 9—Stearic; 10—Nonadecanoic; 11—Nonadecylic; 12—Arachidonic, 13—Docosahexaenoic; 12—Docosatetraenoic. The figures obtained from uninfected molluscs are taken as zero levels. Up—Increase of proportion, down—Decrease of proportion [7].

study the reactions of the liver of molluscs infected with parthenitae of *Sch. turkestanicum* seems a very interesting idea.

In the period between 2009 and 2011, we collected 585 specimens of *L. auricularia* in the bodies of water in the northeastern part of Uzbekistan (Tashkent, Syrdarya and Jizzakh Provinces). To find out the rate of infection with parthenitae and cercariae of *Sch. turkestanicum* in molluscs, we used the method we had developed earlier [49]. We placed every specimen in separate glasses filled with water (50–100 ml) heated to a temperature of 25–30°C. In these conditions, the molluscs were reproducing cercariae for 1–2 hours. The molluscs collected in the bodies of water were divided into age groups, their age having been determined by the size of their shells. Thus, three age groups were formed (from 10.0 mm to 30.0 mm): the "small" (10.0–12.5 mm), "medium-sized" (12.6–15.0 mm) and large (20.0–30.0 mm). Only the members of the "medium-sized" and "large" mollusc groups proved to be infected with *Sch. turkestanicum.* The infected and uninfected (reference) molluscs were used to carry out the histological research.

We used 22 specimens of molluscs *L. auricularia* to carry out the histological research. We cut out the hepatopancreas of live molluscs and put them into 10% neutral formalin and 70% ethylated spirit. To estimate the morphology, we dyed the cut areas with haematoxylin-eosin following the methods of Van Gieson and Mallory [50–52].

We discovered parthenitae and cercariae of one trematode species, *Sch. turkestanicum* in the studied molluscs. In the studied populations of *L. auricularia*, we recorded an average infection rate of ±1.88%. In some biotopes ("The Tashkent Sea", Tashkent Province, 15 June 2009), the infection rate ranged between ±0.5 and ± 3.76% (20 July

2009). In June and July 2010 and 2011, we obtained the same figures, with insignificant deviations.

Only "large" and "medium-sized" specimens of *L. auricularia* in the populations we studied proved to be infected with the parasite.

The morphology of the hepatopancreas in the reference and infected molluscs is given in **Figures 8** and **9**.

Parthenitae and cercariae of *Sch. turkestanicum* were found only in the hepatopancreas of the studied molluscs *L. auricularia.* It means that the hepatopancreas is a common place this trematode lives in (**Figure 9**). Nevertheless, we admit that parthenitae can live in other organs, particularly in heavily infected specimens.

The microscopic inspection of the infected hepatopancreas revealed noticeable changes in its condition. The hepatopancreas (liver) loses its elasticity, becomes friable and increases in size, the last factor caused by the growth of mother and daughter sporocysts. The milky-coloured sporocysts are quite noticeable against the brown of the mollusc's liver: they seem to pierce the liver's parenchyma. The hepatopancreas of the specimens infected with parthenitae and cercariae become greyish-yellow or whitish-green.

The histological research demonstrated that in almost all the cuts parthenitae and cercariae concentrated in the connective tissue of the hepatopancreas. The parasites affect mechanically the connective tissue and acini. The heavily infected molluscs had their lacunar spaces and blood vessels pressed. As a result, degenerative and necrotic changes were observed in the cellular elements of the connective tissue, the fibrillar structures and the main substance. The cores of the connective tissue cells were in most cases highly resistant. When the cells were destroyed, they still remained unchanged in the space between the acini for a long time. Other fibrous structures of the connective tissue were also destroyed. We observed the destruction of the reticular fibres in the space between the acini. The hepatopancreas of heavily infected

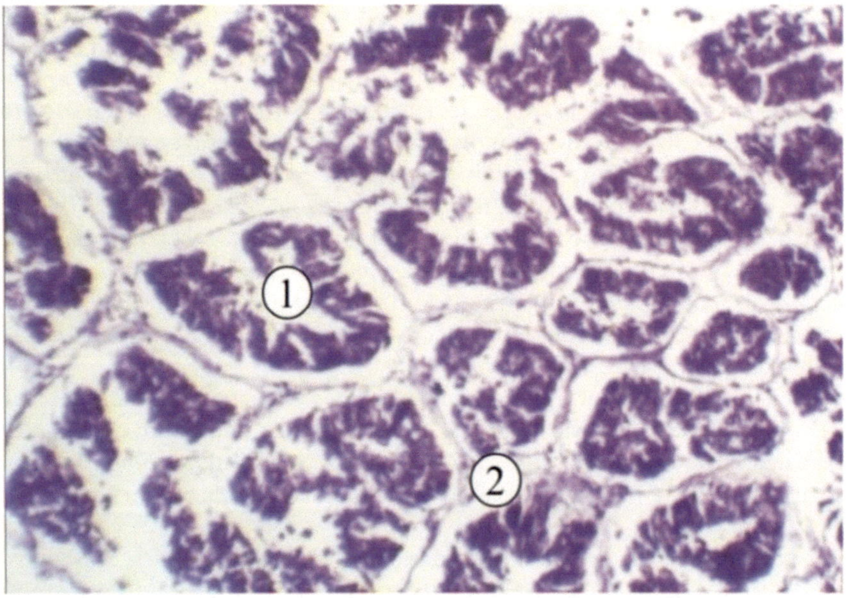

Figure 8.
The microstructure of hepatopancreas Lymnaea auricularia, (control):1—Acinus, 2—Between acinar partition. Objective 10, ocular 10 (original) [7].

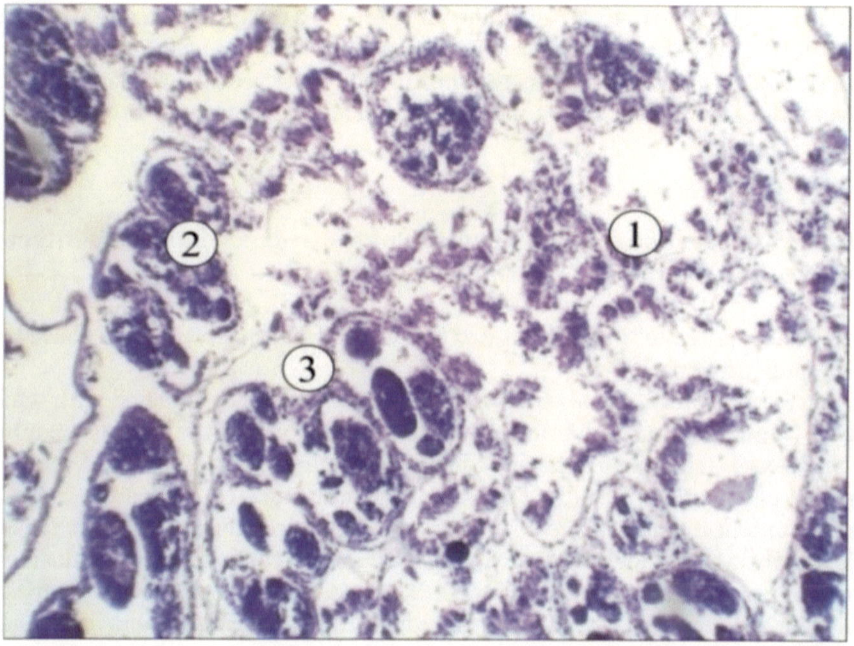

Figure 9.
The microstructure of hepatopancreas Lymnaea auricularia larvae infected Schistosoma turkestanicum. 1—Karyolysis, 2—Karyorrhexis, 3—Pycnosis. Objective 40, ocular 10 (original) [7].

molluscs increased greatly in size. The number of acini decreased considerably. Most of the acini were destroyed.

The parasites concentrating on the central part of the organ force the acini to its periphery, which results in a destruction for most of the acini.

Having destructed the connective tissue between the acini and concentrated there, the parasites pressed the acini. The walls of the acini went nearer to each other, and the space between them became smaller or disappeared at all. The cells that formed the acini's walls deformed, becoming shorter and flatter. The hepatocytes and calcareous cells of hepatopancreas showed signs of autolysis. Degenerative and necrotic processes (pyknosis, karyorrhexis, karyolysis) were observed in the hepatocytes.

We established that the histological structure of the hepatopancreas of the mollusc hosts infected heavily with parthenitae and cercariae of different groups of trematodes changes considerably. The enormous necrotic disintegration of the molluscs' hepatopancreas is accompanied by considerable destructive changes in other organs [18]. The recent research into the influence of parthenitae and cercariae of trematodes from the families Schistosomatidae and Bilharziellidae on the organism of the molluscs and their metabolism has given the same results [45, 53–58].

The pathogenicity of larvae of certain trematode species for the mollusc hosts is an arguable value. It is determined by such changeable factors as the number of parasites specimens in the host and the age and physiological state of the molluscs, as well as their immunological response. However, the factors mentioned above are not sufficient in most cases to prevent the molluscs' infection with trematodes. This is confirmed by the results of the histological research into the organs of molluscs infected with various trematode species. In most cases, scientists recorded considerable changes in the structure and functions of the organs infected with parthenitae and cercariae [18, 19, 41, 45, 59–62]. The same refers to the histopathalogic changes in the hepatopancreas of molluscs *L. auricularia* infected with parthenitae and cercariae of *Sch. turkestanicum*; the changes are conditioned by the pressure the larvae put on the liver tissues and the impact of metabolic product, both from the parasites and the host.

3. Changes in the histological structure of the organs of animals infected with *Schistosoma turkestanicum* Skrjabin, 1913

The issues related to the pathology of this infection in sheep and cattle have been studied quite properly [63–69].

Changes in the histological structure of the organs of sheep infected with schistosomiasis (**Figures 10** and **11**): intestine. Strong hyperaemia of the mucous membrane with occasional stripe-shaped haemorrhages was detected in the course of the inspection of the small intestine. The wall of the intestine is thickened unevenly. The intestine content is liquid mixed with blood and fibrous membranes. When the animal is heavily infected with the trematode, hard nodules and sometimes calcareous deposits appear on the mucous membrane. The nodules may appear on the surface of the mucous membrane individually or in groups, forming stripes 20 cm long. Each nodule is about the size of a poppy seed.

In the course of the histological study, we established that the mucous membrane was slightly oedematous and unevenly infiltrated with leukocytes, which is particularly noticeable near the surface of the mucous membrane and in the places where the helminths' eggs concentrate. Usually, schistosoma's eggs at various stages of development can be found in any layer of the intestine. Some of them do not produce any evident reaction, others cause concentrations of leukocytes, while the third, more mature ones, are enclosed in scar tissue and calcified or surrounded by giant cells.

In the areas of active infiltration, the intestinal villi around the helminth eggs, particularly their tips, are damaged. The epithelial cells in these areas are affected by dystrophy, their protoplasm is slightly coloured by eosin and in places they are completely lysed.

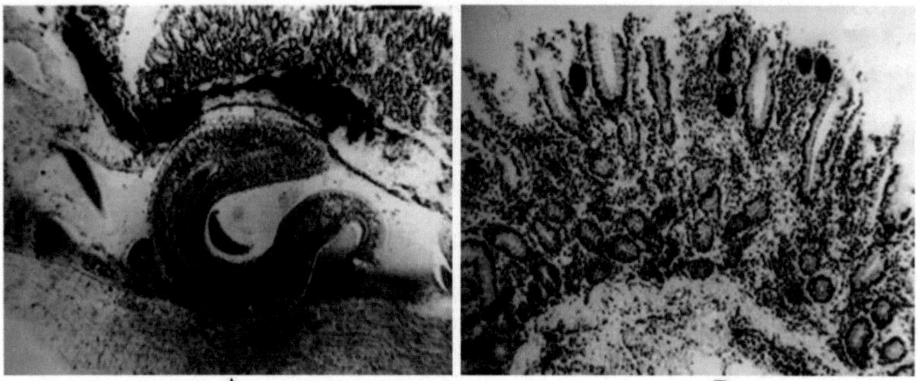

A B

Figure 10.
The small intestine: A—A mature schistosoma specimen is lying in the lumen of a dilated blood vessel (× 25); B—Oedema and the infiltration of the areas filled with eggs with the cellular elements (× 200) [7].

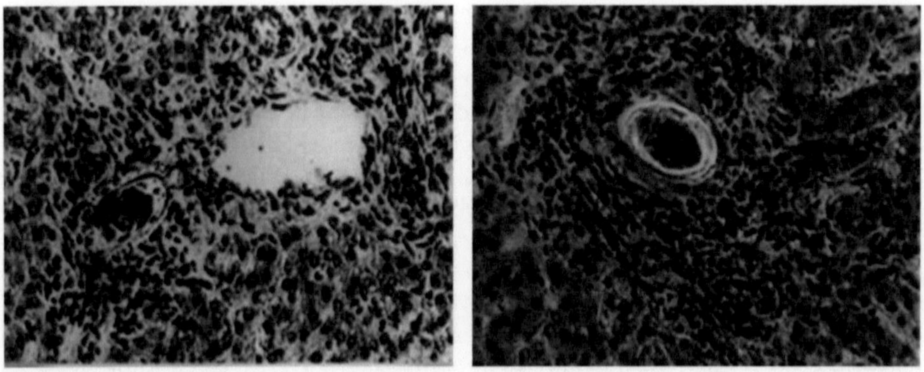

Figure 11.
Liver: A—The penetration of the egg through the vein's wall (× 200); B—A schistosoma egg in the liver parenchyma (× 200) [7].

The surface of the mucous membrane is thickly infiltrated with cell elements consisting of lymphocytes, leukocytes and histiocytes, the most common of which are eosinophils.

The layer under the mucous membrane is oedematous, with dilated blood vessels visible in many places. Bodies of mature schistosoma are visible inside them. Trematodes can be seen in larger vessels cut crosswise and lengthwise. Between their bodies, inside the vessels, are the blood plasma and numerous erythrocytes. The endothelium of such vessels is flattened and often barely visible.

In smaller vessels, the helminths' bodies block the vessels lumina and dilate the walls. In these vessels the parasites cuticle contacts the vessel's endothelium.

The serous layer of the intestine wall is oedematous and much thicker than normal, with slight dilation of the connective tissue and its slight infiltration with lymphoid cells.

In large vessels, the parasites dilate the lumina; smaller vessels are characterised by atrophic changes caused by the parasite's pressing against the vessel wall. The embolised capillaries are characterised by strong proliferative reaction, leading to the formation of productive nodules [68].

The liver is slightly larger than normal. Its surface is smooth, with stripes of pseudomembrane visible on the capsule. Grey-white nodules the size of a poppy seed can be seen under the capsule and in a cut liver. A microscopic examination of these nodules revealed schistosoma eggs with end thorns.

The liver capsule is oedematous and friable and is slightly infiltrated with globocellular lymphocytes. The interlobular connective tissue is slightly thicker than normal and infiltrated with lymphocytic and leukocytic cells. In some places, small haemorrhages could be seen around the vessels and at the edges of the liver lobes.

The liver's blood vessels are dilated, with blood stagnation recorded within them. The central veins are also dilated and contain blood with dark brown iron-bearing pigment. It can also be seen around the vein among the cells of the liver lobes.

The capillaries branching off the central veins are filled with blood.

Nodules with fragments of the helminths or their eggs in the centre could often be seen in the stroma of the interlobular partitions and in the blood vessels or among the liver cells, at the edges of the lobes. Accumulations of cellular elements consisting of eosinophilic and neutrophilic leukocytes, lymphocytes and single disintegrating erythrocytes could be seen around the nodules. The walls of the infected vessels were heavily thinned, the vessels containing inside them the bodies or eggs of the parasites. The nearby bile ducts were thickened and proliferated. The structure of the hepatis tubules changed; the cells were slightly coloured with eosin or were completely necrotised, which was why the contours of the lever cells were hardly visible and their cores were in a state of pyknosis, rhexis and lysis. The necrotic areas are of different size, in places occupying almost half of the liver lobe.

The results of the histological demonstrated that the formation of nodules with concentrations of cellular elements and the weak growth of the connective tissue are the main changes in the liver infected with schistosomiasis. As the pathological process develops, necroses of the liver parenchyma form around the parasitic nodule.

The pancreas. The thickening of the interlobular connective tissue underlines the lobular structure of the pancreas. The tissue is highly swollen and saturated with serous exudate containing moderate quantities of lymphocytes, eosinophils, histiocytes and proliferating connective elements. The blood vessels of the interlobular connective tissue are dilated and filled with blood. Mature parasites can be seen in the lumina of the vessels. Blood plasma and numerous disintegrating erythrocytes can be seen in the lumina of the vessels, between the parasites, and outside them. The walls of such vessels are thinner than normal and ruptured in some places; the endothelium is dense and often hardly visible. Individual small blood vessels are blocked completely by the helminths, which results in the strongly dilated walls. The parasite's cuticle contacts the vessel endothelium.

The structure of the interlobular connective tissue is not so clear. The glandular cells of the pancreas's parenchyma containing the parasite's eggs undergo various necrotic changes. The pancreas's parenchyma is darker and denser, its lobes moved apart. Some of the lobes are atrophied; the lobes' colour is uneven. When observed under high magnification, the lighter lobes demonstrate the development of the connective tissue and atrophy of the glandular zymogenic tissue. The islets of Langerhans can hardly be discerned in such mutated lobes.

The changes in the pancreas described above show that, concentrating on the blood vessels of the interlobular connective tissue, schistosoma cause thromboses of some vessels. Infiltrative and proliferative processes begin around the newly formed thrombi, which leads to a necrosis of the glandular tissue.

The mesentery lymphatic notes are oedematous and larger than normal. The mesenterial vessels are dilated and their walls are thinned. Calcified areas were recorded in the intersected lymphatic nodes.

The lymphatic sini under the capsule and in the centre are dilated and in some places are thickly infiltrated with eosinophilic leukocytes; however, the follicles of the lymphatic nodes remain unchanged, apart from the areas where they are pressed directly by the growing nodules. In these areas, most of the lymphoid tissue is atrophied. They are also somewhat oedematous. The sini are highly dilated and filled with reticular syncytium cells.

As for the other organs, we did not detect any pathological changes in them characteristic of this infection.

The histological studies demonstrate that *Sch. turkestanicum* causes obvious pathologic changes in a number of organs of sheep and goats. The pathological process takes place mostly in the organs' blood system, which is caused by the mature trematodes parasitising them and the migration of the eggs they lay [6, 68].

It should be noted that the principal changes in the liver infected with schistosomiasis consist in the formation of nodules, where the cellular elements accumulate and the connective tissue grows. As the pathologic process develops, areas of liver parenchyma necroses appear around the parasitic nodule.

As for larger blood vessels in the intestine, the parasites dilate their lumina, while in smaller ones they cause atrophic changes associated with the parasite's pressure against their walls.

The areas of the intestine where schistosoma lay their eggs also undergo pathologic changes, characterised by the formation of nodules under the mucous membrane. Penetrating into the small blood vessels of the mucous membrane, the trematode eggs rupture the vessels' walls, which results in inflammatory processes.

The change in the histological structure of the organs of cattle infected with schistosomiasis (**Figures 12–14**): intestine. The infected small intestine is characterised by haemorrhaging areas in its mucous membrane. The intestine content is liquid mixed with blood and fibrous membranes. The wall of the intestine is thickened unevenly, and the space inside the organ is obliterated. Thrombosed veins protrude from the serous membrane. The intestine's mucous membrane is covered with masses of nodules forming stripes that protrude from the walls of the intestine. These nodules may be individual or form groups. The size of each nodule is the same as in sheep. The structure of the nodules is dense, with calcareous deposits. Unevenly dilated blood vessels (veins) filled with thrombi can be observed in different parts of the small intestine. These vessels contain mature schistosoma, which were found there after the dissection.

In the course of the morphological research, we established that the overall structure of the intestine remained unchanged. The mucous membrane of the small intestine contains tissues with deep infiltration of leukocytic cells. The infiltrated areas are in most cases concentrated around the groups of eggs. The intestine's muscular layer remains undamaged, except for ruptures in some small vessels. The structure of the intestinal villi is damaged in the strongly infiltrated areas and around the egg concentrations. The epithelial cells are dystrophic in these areas; their protoplasm is slightly coloured with eosin and is completely lysed in some places. The parts of the intestinal villi that remain are filled with mucus with single or multiple lymphocytes.

In the early phases of the infection, the nodules form only under the mucous membrane of the small intestine. They also spread into the subserous layer. They actually can be found everywhere, mainly, in the areas of the intestine intersected with numerous vessels. The small vessels are filled with the bodies of mature helminths, which block the entire lumen. All the layers of the infected vessel are greatly damaged. The under the endothelial layer layer of the intima is thicker than normal and filled with cellular infiltrate. The contours of the muscle layer become unclear, and fascicles of muscle fibres thicken and begin to grow in various directions, growing into the surrounding connective tissue. The lumina of the vessels are filled with plasma or blood together with the cellular elements. The submucous layer of the mucous membrane is oedematous, with dilated blood vessels visible in many places. The vessels' lumina are filled with the bodies of mature schistosoma. The base of the mucous membrane is infiltrated with lymphoid, histiocytic cells. The bodies of mature helminths are seen in many of the vessels of the mucous membrane intersected crosswise and lengthwise.

The liver is larger than normal; its surface is usually smooth. The organ's lobularity remains unchanged. The surface of the cut resembles marble, which is caused by the thickening of the interlobular partitions. Greyish-white spots can be seen under the capsule in different parts of the liver. These are nodules that are calcified or are in the process of calcification. Their size is that of a poppy seed or larger. These nodules

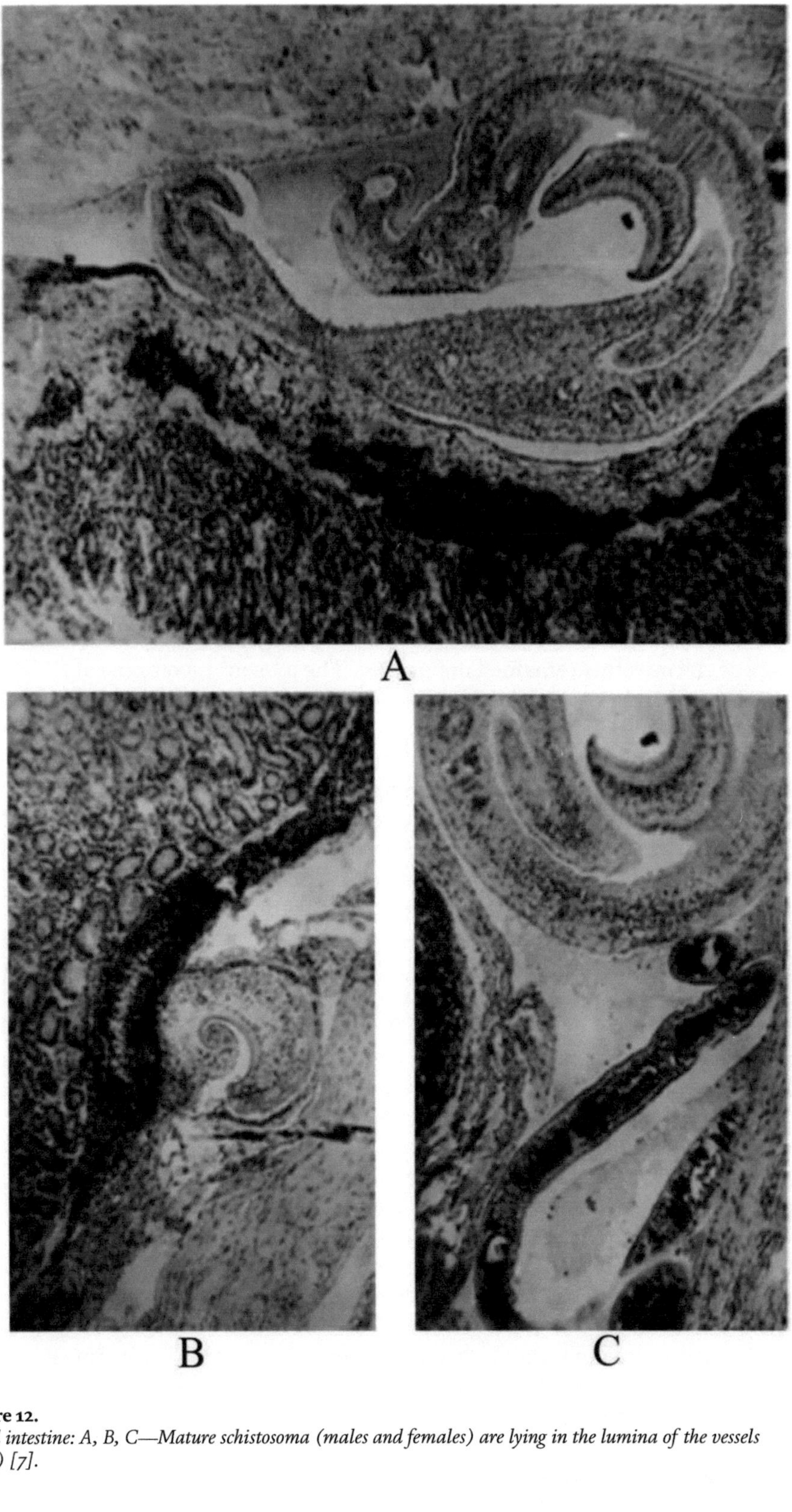

Figure 12.
Small intestine: A, B, C—Mature schistosoma (males and females) are lying in the lumina of the vessels (× 25) [7].

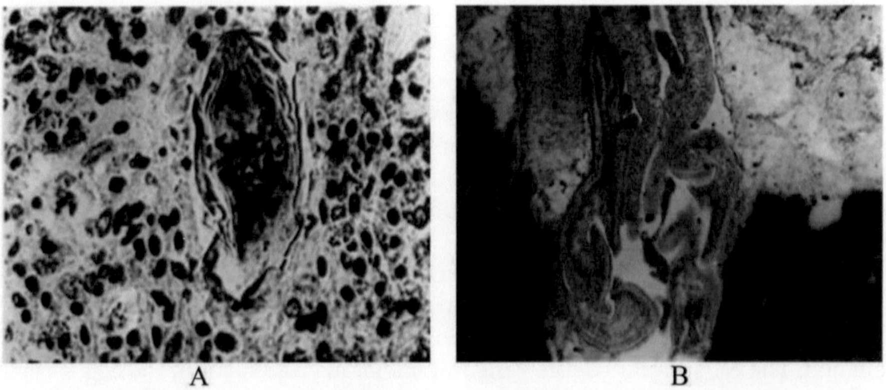

Figure 13.
Pancreas: A—Schistosoma egg in the tissues of the pancreas. The glandular cells undergo dystrophic changes (× 400); B—Mature parasites in the lumina of a blood vessel (× 25) [7].

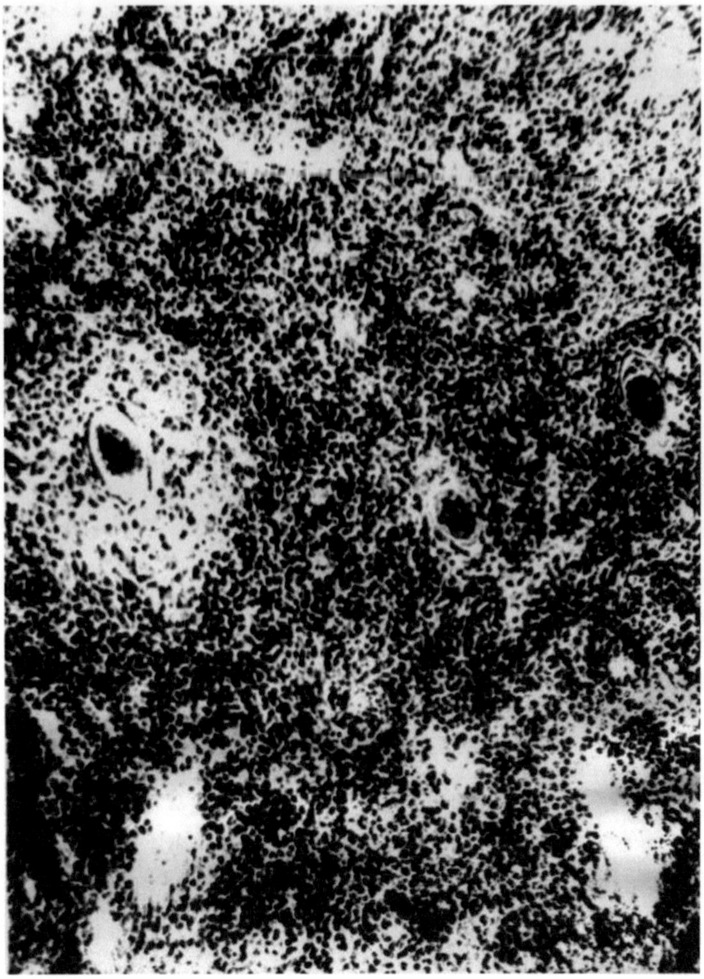

Figure 14.
Lymphatic node: Schistosoma eggs (× 200) [7].

contain schistosoma eggs. Dissected veins release blood with milky-white trematodes *Sch. turkestanicum*. The liver infected by schistosomiasis looks like that affected by nodular cirrhosis.

In the course of the histological study, we established that the lobular structure of the liver remains clear. The interlobular connective tissues are infiltrated with cellular elements. The lumina of the interlobular veins dilate considerably. Together with blood components, it contains the bodies of the parasites, which sometimes block its entire space.

Nodules produced by the migrating *Schistosoma* eggs can be found inside the liver, both in the interlobular layers of the stroma and within the lobes. The egg is oval and elongated, with two thorns, one of which is sharpened and the other has the form of a bent end. The eggs contain developing miracidia. In cross section, the egg is usually round.

Nodules with the eggs of the parasites in the centre can often be found in the stroma of the interlobular partitions, in the blood vessels or among the liver cells. Eosinophilic and neutrophilic leukocytes and lymphocytes accumulate around the eggs. The nodules' structure is not always the same. At early stages, the nodules are cell-like, consisting of clusters of giant cells with gentle connective tissue fibres. As the nodule develops, the egg can lie freely within the former's space, with eosinophilic leukocytes, lymphoid cells and histiocytes accumulating around the latter. Phagocytic cells form around the eggs.

It is interesting to note that some dissections revealed the parasite's eggs in the process of their penetrating through the wall of a vessel.

Changes in the pancreas. The lobular structure of the pancreas is obvious because of the dilation of the interlobular connective tissue. The latter is swollen and oedematous and is saturated with serous exudates, which includes lymphocytes, eosinophils, histiocytes, proliferating connective elements and small quantities of nuclear fragments having the form of scattered chromatin bodies.

The blood vessels of the interlobular connective tissue are dilated and filled with blood. The bodies of the mature parasites can be found laying in the lumina of some vessels. Blood plasma and numerous disintegrating erythrocytes are seen in the vessels' lumina, between the parasites, and outside them. The walls of such vessels are thinner than normal and ruptured in places; their endothelium is dense and barely discernible. Some small-diameter vessels are blocked completely with the bodies of the parasites, which is why their wall is heavily stretched. In such vessels, the parasite's cuticle contacts the vessel's endothelium. The structure of the interlobular connective tissue in the vast areas around the affected vessels is unclear and is replaced by adipose tissue, which has the form of cavities consisting of multiple cells. The glandular cells of the organ's parenchyma with the eggs of the parasites undergo various dystrophic changes: pyknosis, rhexis and lysis.

The pancreas's parenchyma is smaller and denser than usual, and its glands are moved apart and have a darker colour than in normal tissue. Some lobes close to the affected areas are heavily atrophied and have uneven colouring. Under high magnification we can see that the lighter lobes are characterised by the development of connective tissue and atrophy of the glandular zymogenic tissue.

The lymphatic nodes. The mesentery lymphatic nodes are oedematous and slightly enlarged. Calcified nodules can be seen in an intersected infected node, which is connected with the presence of schistosoma eggs.

The histological examination showed that the lymphatic sini were dilated and in some places infiltrated strongly with eosinophilic leukocytes. The lymphatic follicular

DOI: http://dx.doi.org/10.5772/intechopen.109876

tissue remains unchanged, except for the sections where it is pressed directly by the nodules. In these areas, most of the active lymphoid tissue is oedematous or lost. The sini are dilated and filled with various wandering cells from the reticular syncytium. The presence of the typical *Schistosoma* eggs in the centre of the nodule's accounts for the damage cause.

The helminths staying for a long time inside the blood vessels cause inflammatory processes, which leads to the formation of thrombi. In its turn, this results in the development of chronic oedema, metabolic malfunction and necroses in different organs. The eggs emitted by trematode females penetrate into small veins and embolise them. The dense eggshell and the sharp thorn of the egg traumatise the vascular wall and cause inflammation. The inflammation is of an ordinary productive character, causing the growth of the tissular elements or the diffusive destruction of the organ's stroma. As the pathological process develops, the organ's parenchyma undergoes atrophic and degenerative changes, which finally leads to necrosis [3, 5, 67]. Thus, it is obvious that *Schistosoma* belong to highly pathogenic trematode species causing strong changes in the organism of an infected animal.

Author details

Djalaliddin A. Azimov, Firuza D. Akramova, Alisher A. Safarov and Erkin B. Shakarboev
Institute of Zoology of the Academy of Sciences of the Republic of Uzbekistan, Tashkent, Uzbekistan

*Address all correspondence to: safarov-alisher@mail.ru

References

[1] Kennedy K. Ecological parasitology. Moscow: Mir; 1978. p. 280

[2] Shakarboyev EB. The Ecological and Functional Interrelations of *Orientobilharzia Turkestanica* (Skrjabin, 1913)—*Bos taurus* Linnaeus, 1758 in the Parasite-Host System: A PhD Thesis in Biology. Tashkent: Institute of Zoology; 1996. p. 134

[3] Azimov DA. Tremadodes—Parasites of Animals and Human. Tashkent: Mehnat; 1986. p. 128

[4] Azimov DA. The diagnosis of orientobilharziasis. In: The Materials of the Conference Dedicated to the Memory of N.V. Badanin. Tashkent: Fan; 1968. pp. 33-36

[5] Azimov DA. On the habitats of trematodes from the genus Orientobilharzia. The Uzbek Biological Journal. Tashkent: Science. 1978;**3**:44-46

[6] Azimov DA, Arifjanov ZK. The environmental conditions as the main factors of the distribution of *Orientobilharzia turkestanica* and the formation of infection nidi. The Bulletin of All-Russian Skrjabin Scientific Research Institute of Helmonthology. 1969;**2**:5-7

[7] Azimov DA, Akramova FD, Shakarboyev EB, Norqobilov BT, Shakarbayev UA, Sayitqulov BS. Schistosomiasis of Animals. Tashkent: Fan; 2019. p. 320

[8] Sidorov VS, Vysotskaya RU, Smirnov LP, Guryanova SD. The Comparative Biochemistry of Helminths of Fish: Amino Acids, Proteins, Lipids. Leningrad: Nauka; 1989. p. 240

[9] Lizenko YI. The Lipid Composition of the Gonads of Large Whitefish in the Lakes of Karelia (Lake Onega Basin). The Biochemistry of Freshwater Fish of Karelia. Petrozavodsk: Science; 1980. pp. 15-21

[10] Yuneva TV, Schepkina AM, Shulman GY, Melnikov VV. The lipid composition of zvezduziid from the equatorial Atlantic. The Hydrobiological Magazine. 1992;**28**(5):61-67

[11] Kreps YM. The Lipids of the Cellular Membranes. Leningrad: Nauka; 1981. p. 340

[12] Zengbush P. Molecular and cellular biology. Moscow: Medicine; 1982. p. 438

[13] Sidorov VS. The ecological biochemistry of fish. In: Lipids. Leningrad: Nauka; 1983. p. 240

[14] Shakarboyev EB, Azimov DA. The biochemical aspects of the adaptation of trematode *Orientobilharzia turkestanica* (Skrjabin, 1913) to its habitat's conditions. In: Reports by the Academy of Sciences of the Republic of Uzbekistan. Tashkent: Science; 1997. pp. 43-46

[15] Oymatov M, Shakarbayev EB. The fatty-acid composition of the phospholipids in the liver of cows *Bos taurus* infected with trematode *Orientobilharzia turkestanica*. The Magazine of the Evolutionary Biochemistry and Physiology. 2000;**1**(36):30-32

[16] Christie JD, Foster WB, Stauber LA. The effect of parasitism and starvation on carbohydrate reserves of *Biomphalaria glabrata*. Journal of Invertebrate Pathology. 1974;**22**(1):55-62

[17] Stadnichenko AP. On the change of the blood protein composition in

Lymnaea stagnalis (L.) connected with age. The Hydrobiological Magazine. 1970;**2**(6):124-127

[18] Stadnichenko AP. On the pathogenic impact of trematode larvae on *Viviparus viviparus* (L., 1758) (Gastropoda, Prosobranchia). Parasitology. 1972;**VI**(2):154-160

[19] Stadnichenko AP. The rate of infection with parthenitae *Bucephalus polymorphus* baer (trematodes) in *Unio pictorum* and *Anodonta piscinalis* (Mollusca, Lamellibranchia) and the parasites' impact on the hosts' organisms. Parasitology. 1974;**VIII**(5):420-425

[20] Aruna K, Simba SS. Comparative studies on protein contents of the hepatopancreas of infected freshwater snails. *Melanoides tuberculatus* (Muller) and *Indoplanorbis exustus* (Deshayee). Comparison of the Physiology, Ecology. 1989;**14**(2):83-87

[21] Dembitsky VM. The plasmagenous composition of the phospholipid classes of different organs and tissues of octopus octopus sp. The Magazine for the Evolution of Biochemistry and Physiology. 1981;**XVII**(3):296-298

[22] Kostetsky YE, Shipunov YA. The evolution of the phospholipids content of marine invertebrates. The Magazine for the Evolution of Biochemistry and Physiology. 1983;**XIX**(1):11-19

[23] Kostetsky YE. The phospholipid composition of molluscs and Crustacea. The Biology of the Sea. 1985;**2**:52-61

[24] Kostetsky YE, Sergeyuk NN. Phospholipids and their plasmologen forms in the muscular tissue of marine invertebrates. The Magazine for the Evolution of Biochemistry and Physiology. 1985;**XXXI**(3):235-298

[25] Kostetsky YE, Sergeyuk NN. The impact of seasonal factors on the phospholipids content and their plasmologen forms in the muscular tissue of marine invertebrates. The Magazine for the Evolution of Biochemistry and Physiology. 1986;**XXII**(2):132-142

[26] Almatov KT. The Mechanisms of the Development of Damages in the Mitochondria and the Role of the Steatolytic System. The Abstract of a Doctoral Thesis. Tashkent: Institute of Biochemistry; 1990. p. 32

[27] Lizenko YI, Vinyatsinsky VF, Sidorov VS, Klepkina MN. The Change of Lysolecithin Content in Carps Infected with Various Diseases. The Biochemistry of Young Specimens of Freshwater Fish. Petrozavodsk: Science; 1985. pp. 33-39

[28] Guryanova SD. The Impact of Dactyeogyrus Sp. Monogenes on the Lipid Composition of some Tissues. In: The Biochemistry of Young Fish in the Winter Period. Petrozavodsk: Science; 1987. pp. 102-106

[29] Saatov TS, Zaynutdinov BR. Phospholipid metabolism in some pathological conditions. In: The Ukrainian Biochemical Magazine. 1984;**56**:285-293

[30] Khochachka P, Semero J. In: The Strategy of Biochemical Adaptation. Moscow: Mir; 1977. p. 390

[31] Alekseyenko AV. The role of the lipids and the products of peroxidation in the biosynthesis and functional activity of DNA. In: The Biochemistry of Lipids and their Role in Metabolism. Moscow: Medicine; 1981. pp. 3-16

[32] Petrov RV, Ataullakhanov RI. Cellular Membranes and Immunity. Moscow; 1991. p. 144

[33] Marzoyeva AI, Andryushchenko AP, Vladimirov YA. Thyroid hormones

and the activity of mitochondrial phospholipase in the liver of rats. The Bulletins of the Experimental Biology and Medicine. 1983;**12**:45-46

[34] Kuzmina VV, Pomazanskaya LF, Zabelinsky SA, Pustovoy YK. The fatty-acid composition of the lipids in the mucous membrane of the intestine of freshwater bony fish. The Magazine for the Evolution of Biochemistry and Physiology. 1982;**XVIII**(6):558-563

[35] Kotyk A, Yanachek K. The Membranous Transport. Moscow: Mir; 1980. p. 314

[36] Arkhipov AV. The change of the lipid metabolism of hens in ontogenesis. The Agricultural Biology. 1980;**30**(5):756-761

[37] Nefedova ZA. The change of fixed fatty acids in the early ontogenesis of some fish species. In: The Biochemistry of Ecto- and Endoteric Organisms. Petrozavodsk: Science; 1989. pp. 53-60

[38] Ginetsinskaya TA. Trematodes, their Life Cycles, Biology and Evolution. L: Nauka; 1968. p. 411

[39] Kruglov ND. Molluscs from the pond snail family (Lymnaeidae, Gastropoda, Pulmonata). In: Europe and North Asia. Smolensk: Published by SGPU; 2005. p. 507

[40] James BI. The effects of parasitism by larval Digenea on the digestive gland of the intertidal prosobranch, Littorinasaxatilis (Olivi) subsp. tenebrosa (Montagu). Parasitology. 1965;**55**(1):93-115

[41] Sluiters JF. Development of *Trichobilharzia ocellata* in *Lymnaea stagnalis* and the effects of infection on the reproductive system of the host. Z. Parasitenk. 1981;**64**(3):303-319

[42] Stadnichenko AP. Interrelations in the "host (freshwater mollusc)—Parasite (trematodes)" system. The Hydrobiological Magazine. 1984;**15**(6):31-36

[43] Cheng TC, James HA. The histopathology of *Credodistomum* sp. infection in the second intermediate host, *Sphaerium striatinum*. Proceedings of the Helminthological Society of Washington. 1960;**27**:67-68

[44] Azimov DA. The Schistosomes of Animals and Humans. Tashkent: Fan; 1975. p. 152

[45] Horak P, Kolářova L, Adema CM. Biology of the Schistosoma genus Trichibilharzia. In: Advances in Parasitology. 2002;**52**:156-233

[46] Shakarboyev EB. Trematodes of the Vertebrates of Uzbekistan (the Species Composition, Circulation Ways, Ecology Ad Biology): A Doctoral Thesis in Biology. Tashkent: Institute of Zoology; 2009. p. 243

[47] Akramova FD, Shakarboyev EB, Golovanov VI, Isakova DT, Azimov DA. The life cycle of trematode *Dendritobilharzia loossi* (Schistosomatida, Bilharziellidae), parasite of aquatic birds. The Bulletin of Zoology. 2007;**6**(41):511-520

[48] Akramova FD. Trematodes Bilharziellidae; their Origin and Evolution: A Doctoral Thesis. Tashkent: Institute of Zoology; 2011. p. 229

[49] Shakarbaev UA, Akramova FD, Khakberdiyeva DM. The reaction of the tissues of *Lymnaea auricularia* to developing larvae of *Orientobilharzia turkestanica* (Skrjabin, 1913). In: Biology, the Science of the 21st Century: The 15th International Pushchino School-Conference of Young Dcholars. Pushchino. 2011. 18-22 April. A Collection of Theses. Pushchino: Nauka; 2011. p. 201

[50] Romeys B. Microscopic technique. Moscow: Medicine; 1953. p. 708

[51] Merkulov GA. The Course of the Pathohistological Technique. Leningrad: Medicine; 1969. p. 422

[52] Volkova OV, Yeletsky YK. The Principles of Histology with the Histological Technique. Moscow: Science; 1971. p. 259

[53] Patnaik MM, Ray SK. A histopathologic study of Lymnaea auricularia var. rufescens infected wirh larval stages of *Echinostoma revolutum*. Japanese Journal of Medical Science and Biology. 1960;**19**:44-56

[54] Morand S, Manning SD, Woolhouse MEJ. Parasite-host coevolution and geographic patterns of parasite infectivity and host susceptibility. Proceedings of the Royal Society of London Series B—Biological Sciences. 1996;**263**:119-128

[55] Sapp KK, Loker ES. A comparative study of mechanisms underlying digenean-snail specificity: in vitro interactions between hemocytes and digenean larvae. Journal of Parasitology. 2000;**86**:1020-1029

[56] Zhang SM, Leonard PM, Adema CM, Loker ES. Parasite responsive IgSF members in the snail Biomphalaria glabrata: Characterization of novel genes with tandemly arranged IgSF domains and a fibrinogen domain. Immunogenetics. 2001;**53**:684-694

[57] Hahn UK, Bender RC, Bayne CJ. Involvement of nitric oxide in killing of *Schistosoma mansoni* sporocysts by haemocytes from resistant Biomphalaria glabrata. Journal of Parasitology. 2001;**87**:778-785

[58] Russo J, Lagadic L. Effects of parasitism and pesticide exposure on charac teristics and functions of hemocyte populations in the freshwater snail *Lymnaea palustris* (Gastropoda, Pulmonata). Cell Biology and Toxicology. 2000;**16**:15-30

[59] Cheng TC, Snyder RW. Studies on host—parasite relationships between larval trematodes and their hosts. I. a review. The utilization of the host's glycogen by the intramolluscan larvae of Glypthelmins pennsylvaniensis Cheng and associated phenomena. Transactions of the American Microscopical Society. LXXXI. 1962;**3**:209-288

[60] Stadnichenko AP, Ivanenko LD, Kolosenko NA, Bubon AB, Litvinchuk RV. The pathomorphological changes in the cellular elements of the hemolymph of freshwater pulmonate and prosobranch gastropods infected with trematode parthenitae. Parasitology. 1981;**XV**(5. L.):407-414

[61] Stadnichenko AP, Bubon AB, Litvinchuk RV. The pathomorphological changes in the blood corpuscles of the hemolymph of freshwater molluscs (Bivalvia, Unionidae, Anodontinae) infected with trematode parthenitae. Parasitology. 1983;**XVII**(1. L.):18-23

[62] Avanesyan AV. The Influence of the Molluscs' Defense Reaction on the Development of Trematode Parthenitae (with the Family Echinostomatidae Used as an Example): The Thesis of PhD in Biology. St. Petersburg: Institute of Zoology; 2002. p. 81

[63] MacHattie C. A preliminary note on the life history of *Schistosoma turkestanicum* Skrjabin, 1913. Transactions of Royal Society of Tropical Medicine and Hygiene. 1936;**30**:115-124

[64] Lavrov LI, Vsevolodov BP. Materials on the pathomorphology

of orientobilharziasis of cattle. The Materials of a Scientific Conference. 1966;**Part 2**:120-122

[65] Lavrov LI, Vsevolodov BP. Materials on the pathomorphology of orientobilharziasis of cattle. Helminths and helminthiases of animals of Kazakhstan. Works by the Institute of Zoology under the Academy of Sciences of the Republic of Kazakhstan. 1967;**27**:156-168

[66] Azimov DA, Nurmukhamedov KN. Orientobilharziasis in ruminants. The Agriculture of Uzbekistan. 1967;**7**:56

[67] Azimov DA, Nurmukhamedov KN. New data on the biology of trematode *Orientobilharzia turkestanica* (Schistosomatidae). In: The Zoological Journal. 1968;**10**:1471-1478

[68] Azimov DA, Nurmukhamedov KN. The pathomorphology of orientobilharziasis of sheep and goats. In: The Collection of Works on Helminthology Dedicated to the 90th Anniversary of K.I. Skrjabin. Moscow: Science; 1971. pp. 5-11

[69] Zakhryalov YN. *Orientobilharzia turkestanica* Skrjabin, 1913 Dutt and Srivastava, 1955 in the Far East: The Abstract of a Doctoral Thesis. Alma-Ata: Institute of Zoology; 1975. p. 43

Chapter 6

The Epizootology of Schistosomiasis of Animals

Djalaliddin A. Azimov, Bakhrom T. Norkobilov, Firuza D. Akramova and Ulugbek A. Shakarbaev

Abstract

Among animal schistosomiasis, schistosomiasis caused by *Sch. turkestanicum* is the most common in many countries of Asia and Europe. This chapter highlights the features of the epizootic process of schistosomiasis in domestic animals (sheep, goats, cattle, camels, horses) in Uzbekistan. Stationary foci of animal schistosomiasis are located in the lower reaches of the Amu Darya River—in the farms of Karakalpakstan and the Khorezm region, where the infection rate of cattle, sheep and horses reaches from 18.7 to 43.7%. Sporadic cases of schistosomiasis in small and large cattle were also noted in the farms of North-Eastern Uzbekistan. There was also a significant distribution of *Sch. turkestanicum* among mammals in the post-Soviet countries (Azerbaijan, Kazakhstan, Kyrgyzstan, Turkmenistan and Russia) and other countries of the world (Mongolia, China, Iraq, Iran, India, Pakistan, Turkey, France, Hungary, etc.). Materials are presented for the forecast of the occurrence of schistosomiasis in animals in the zones of development, irrigation and watering of lands.

Keywords: epizootology, schistosomiasis, *Sch. Turkestanicum*, foci, prognosis, stationary

1. The Epizootology of Schistosomiasis of Animals

The epizootology of schistosomiasis is closely connected with the biology of the parasite causing the disease. Hence, the multiplicity of interconnected and interdependent links of the epizootologic chain, on the one hand, is formed by the definitive and intermediate hosts and, on the other hand, by favourable environmental factors. With schistosoma and their hosts present, the cycle of the former is determined by the environment, in particular, by the climate, hydrology and relief of the region they inhabit.

The epizootology of schistosomiasis of animals has been studied in all regions of Uzbekistan stage by stage. The materials are under discussion with the involvement of literary data from local and foreign researchers on schistosomiasis of animals.

The role of molluscs, the intermediate hosts in the distribution of schistosomiasis. The distribution of schistosomiasis both in Uzbekistan and in other countries is connected with the habitat of the intermediate hosts, freshwater molluscs from the family Lymnaeidae, mainly *Lymnaea auricularia*.

We would like to note two factors important from the epizootological aspects: 1) the appearance of molluscs with cercariae in June exposes animals to the infection with schistosoma in the middle of the pasturing season, and 2) the highest infection rate among molluscs and the emission of the largest number of mature cercariae take place in summer-early autumn, which leads to a large number of animals infected with trematodes during the whole of the warm season.

The ear molluscs in the northwestern and northeastern parts of Uzbekistan, the regions with high rates of infection with schistosomiasis, form stable populations of parasites. Emitting a large number of cercariae, these molluscs cause high concentrations of infecting elements near bodies of water, which lead to a rapid spread of infection among the definitive hosts. In addition, moving from one body of water to another, the infected molluscs distribute.

There are a number of works by local and foreign scientists on the role of molluscs in the distribution of schistosomiasis: Dutt, Srivastava (1964), Uvaliyeva, Panin, Lavrov (1968), Stepanov (1969), Kumar (1973); Massoud (1973), Zakhryalov (1975), Sahba et al. (1979), Tang et al. (1983), Azimov (1986), Liu et al. (1987), Athari et al. (1990, 2006), Sakarboyev (1996, 2009), Wang et al. (2000, 2002), Kojabayev (2001), Qiu et al. (2008), Majoros et al. (2010).

The distribution of schistosomiasis. The information on *Sch. turkestanicum* is diverse, which means the problem has been studied properly in some of the regions of our country and around the world.

To analyse and generalise the data we used information on the distribution of *Sch. turkestanicum* around the world.

Taking into account the diversity of the landscapes, climate and economy in different regions of Uzbekistan, on the one hand, and the necessity to concretise the epizootic situation about the disease, on the other hand, we thought it expedient to consider the distribution of the infection in every country.

The Republic of Uzbekistan. In effort to facilitate the analysis and consideration of the impact of the landscapes, climate and economic situation in different regions on the distribution of schistosomiasis, we decided to divide these regions into major areas following the pattern proposed by Akramov et al. (1967).

I. Northeastern Uzbekistan consists of three provinces—Syrdarya, Jizzakh and Tashkent. In this area, schistosoma was recorded in cattle, in pastures on the flood plain of the Syrdarya River and in newly cultivated territories in Syrdarya and Jizzakh provinces [1].

II. Eastern Uzbekistan (Andizhan, Namangan and Fergana provinces). No schistosoma was recorded in this area.

III. Central Uzbekistan (Samarkand, Navoi and Bukhara provinces) occupies a vast territory occupying over one third of the country's area. No schistosoma populations were recorded in animals in this region.

IV. Southern Uzbekistan (Surkhandarya and Kashkadarya provinces). No schistosoma was recorded.

V. North-western Uzbekistan (Republic of Karakalpakstan, Khorezm Province) lying in the lower course of the Amudarya. This is the largest region occupying 42% of the country's area. We were the first to carry out a regular inspection of animals for schistosomiasis [2]. We implemented a comprehensive research programme in the region and recorded a high infection rate in cattle, sheep and goats (**Table 1**).

The data in the table indicate the extensive character of infection with *Sch. turkestanicum* in animals in the natural biocoenoses of northwestern Uzbekistan. The infection rate varied depending on the animal species. So, the rate of infection in cattle was 43.7%, in sheep—20.9%, in goats—12.2%, in camels—8.3%, in horses—18.7%, in donkeys—8.3%, in pigs (domestic)—5.0% and in cats—7.6%. The figures on the rate of infection in wild animals we examined were the following: saigas—12.1%, boars (wild)—17.6% and rats—11.7%. Schistosomiasis and deaths of livestock caused by this disease have been recorded in the Republic of Karakalpakstan and Khorezm Province since 1965. In September-November 1984 and in 2005 scientists recorded outbreaks of invasion in the cattle of Muynak, Kungrad, Kegeyli, Chimbay and Bozatau Districts of the Republic of Karakalpakstan, which resulted in numerous deaths among the animals. Hundreds of thousands of the parasites were found in the dissected animals. The disease is recorded sporadically at other farms of Republic of Karakalpakstan and Khorezm Province.

The recorded infection rate in Khorezm was 18.0% in sheep and 37.7% in cattle. The rate of infection in Karakalpakstan is much higher, with 22.0% of sheep and 46.5% of cattle being parasitised. At some farms, the rate of infection in sheep reaches 30.0% and in cattle 65.0%. We referred these vast regions to those with intense schistosomiasis situation.

Having established the level of distribution of schistosomiasis, we examined carefully the infection's seasonal and age dynamics in the sheep and cattle of this region of Uzbekistan.

According to our research, schistosoma tend to parasitise cattle and sheep of different age groups in all seasons of the year.

Animal species	Animal specimens inspected, total	Infected		Maximal infection rate
		Quantity	%	
Cattle	1450	635	43.7	123,636
Sheep	1175	246	20.9	13,285
Goats	49	6	12.2	65
Camels	12	1	8.3	135
Saigas	33	4	12.1	937
Horses	133	25	18.7	850
Donkeys	12	1	8.3	103
Domestic pigs	20	1	5.0	87
Wild boars	17	3	17.6	543
Domestic dogs	15	—	—	—
Domestic cats	13	1	7.6	23
Pest rats	17	2	11.7	59

Table 1.
The rate of infection with schistosoma in the animals of Uzbekistan (based on full and partial dissection).

The infection dynamics in sheep is mostly the same as that in cattle. The infection curve has one top, with maxima in autumn and winter.

The rate of infection with schistosoma in sheep does not vary greatly depending on the animals' age and the season. The infection dynamics in sheep is as follows: in young sters—69.0% in spring, 67.5% in summer, 70.5% in autumn and 71.0 in winter; in adult animals: 50.0% in spring, 42.0% in summer, 44.0% in autumn and 42.0% in winter.

The following fluctuations were recorded in the youngsters of cattle infected with schistosoma: 93.0% in spring, 70.5% in summer, 90.0 in autumn and 96.0% in winter; animals more than 3 years old: 80.0% in spring and summer, 84.0% in autumn and 86.0% in winter; calves younger than 1 year old also demonstrate increase of the infection rate starting from autumn (12.0–20.0%), with maxima in autumn and winter (64.0%).

In general, the rate of infection in animals remains the same throughout the year, with slight fluctuations depending on the season. From spring to summer, the rate drops a little, and rises starting from autumn, reaching its maximum in winter.

The materials on the distribution of schistosomiasis among the synanthropic (cattle and sheep) animals of the northeastern part of Uzbekistan allow us to refer the region to the areas with an unstable schistosomiasis situation. We suppose that the area is characterised by the spread of the disease and stabilisation of the 'parasite-host' system.

Therefore, schistosomiasis in Uzbekistan depends on the climate and landscapes with necessary biological prerequisites for the completion of individual phases of the parasites ontogenesis. We consider that these prerequisites are provided by the areas in the lower course of the Amudarya and the middle course of the Syrdarya, that is, by the northwestern and northeastern regions of Uzbekistan. The whole complex of proper conditions allowed the parasite to cover a wide range of hosts to circulate in the biocoenoses of the abovementioned regions, which occupy a vast area of Uzbekistan.

In the northwestern part of the country alone schistosoma have been recorded in 12 species of wild and domestic mammals belonging to 6 families. Five of the species, the saiga, Bukhara deer, gazelle, wild boar and schort - tailed rat, were recorded as the trematode's definitive hosts for the first time.

Analysing the obtained materials we could distinguish three areas in Uzbekistan by the degree of infection with schistosomiasis—epizootic, threatened and stable.

The epizootic area covers a large territory including the Republic of Karakalpakstan and Khorezm, Tashkent and Syrdarya provinces. The area features the most favourable conditions for the development of ear pond snails and is inhabited by a large number of these molluscs.

The area under study has all the components of the parasitic system for the circulation of the infection: the parasite—the carrier—the sensitive animals plus suitable ecology.

The threatened area does not feature animals bearing the parasites, but it is inhabited by molluscs, schistosoma's intermediate hosts. It covers the territories of Jizzakh, Surkhandarya, Kashkadarya, Samarkand, Bukhara, Navoi, Fergana, Andizhan and Namangan Provinces. This area may turn into an epizootic one if animals carrying the parasite appear here.

The stable area occupies a considerable portion of deserts, semi-deserts and high mountains. These territories are not inhabited with schistosoma's intermediate hosts and, therefore, have no infected animals [3]. In this work, we also provide data on schistosomiasis in other countries.

Kyrgyzstan. M.G. Toktouchkova (1971) recorded schistosomiasis in the cattle of the Issyk Kul depression. The rate of infection was 1.3%, each animal having been parasitised with 14–400 individuals of schistosoma.

Turkmenistan. D.F. Stepanov (1968–1970) inspected a large number of synanthropic animals for schistosomiasis. The infection is rather common for the cattle and sheep of the Dashoguz oasis. The total rate of infection was 40.3% in cattle and 12.6% in sheep. Schistosomiasis was recorded in 6 districts of the oasis. The highest infection rate in cattle was recorded in Dashoguz Province—62.5%.

Actually, schistosomiasis was recorded in animals in all seasons of the year. The maximal infection rate was recorded in autumn and winter, with some decrease in spring and summer [3].

The materials on the spread of schistosomiasis among the synanthropic animals of Turkmenistan and the relatively high infection rate in the cattle and sheep of Dashoguz Province allow us to refer this region of the country to areas with intense schistosomiasis situations, like some of the regions of Uzbekistan.

On the basis of the facts about the distribution of schistosomiasis among the wild and synanthropic animals of Central Asia given above we distinguish the following groups of areas: 1) areas with high infection rate in synanthropic and wild animals—Uzbekistan; 2) areas with high infection rate in domestic animals—Turkmenistan; 3) areas with relatively low rate of infection in domestic animals—Kyrgyzstan.

Russia (the Far East). The area includes Primorsky and Khabarovsk krais, Amur, Magadan and Sakhalin Provinces and Yakutia.

For the first time, the animals of the Far East were inspected for schistosomiasis by the 60th Union Helminthological Expedition headed by K.I. Skrjabin in 1928. *Sch. bomfordi*, one of the parasites causing schistosomiasis, was found in sheep.

Many years later, P.G. Oshmarin (1963) recorded schistosomiasis in the sheep and cattle of the Far East. The rate of infection in sheep was 6.4% and 20.5% in cattle. Some of the animals were recorded to die due to this disease. K.G. Abramov (1963) reported about *Sch. turkestanicum* found in the blood of the elks of the Amur River area.

Ya.N. Zakhryalov (1964–1975) carried out comprehensive research into schistosomiasis of animals in the Far East. The researcher inspected 8137 animals (7482 specimens of cattle, 394 sheep, 136 horses, 104 pigs, 20 reindeer and 1 goat) and found *Sch. turkestanicum* in the cattle, horses and sheep of the upper and middle Amur areas and in Primorsky. The scientist established that the infection was widely spread in the Far East. In Primorye, the infection rate was 22.9% in cattle and 6.5% in sheep; in the upper Amur area—19.7% in cattle, 30.8% in sheep and 25.0% in horses; in the middle Amur area—6.6% in cattle. In the Far East, schistosoma are distributed over a vast territory, which is conditioned, in Ya.N. Zakhryalov's opinion, by the existence of a dense network of bodies of water in this territory.

Ya.N Zakhryalov (1964, 1972, 1975) studied the age and seasonal dynamics of schistosomiasis in the cattle of the upper Amur area and in Primorsky. The researcher noted that, unlike in Uzbekistan, Kazakhstan and Iran, the age dynamics of the infection in cattle is very strong. The infection rate and the number of the parasites in cattle specimens grow from the age of 5 months to the age of 3 years (0.5–2.6% in calves, 9.8–16.2% in specimens over 1 year old and 30.5–34.4% in adults). Adult animals, from 3 to 18 years old, did not demonstrate any noticeable rise or drop in the infection rate. The scientist refers the age and seasonal dynamics of schistosomiasis to biological factors and specific local economic factors.

Thus, it should be noted that in the territory of the Far East specific animal species—the elk, reindeer and Siberian roe deer—participate in the cycle of schistosomiasis as its definitive hosts. The significant rate of infection among the synanthropic animals and the involvement of wild animals in the circulation of schistosomiasis indicate the specific epizootic schistosomiasis situation in the Far East.

The highly intense schistosomiasis situation in the biocoenoses of domestic and wild (to a lesser extent) animals creates possibilities for the disease to spread over a vast territory of Russia's Far East.

Kazakhstan. Over a century ago, in 1909, K.I. Skrjabin, working as a veterinarian in the present-day city of Jambul, Kazakhstan, discovered a parasite in the branching of the portal vein of cattle, which, when studied carefully, turned out to be a new blood fluke species. In 1913, Skrjabin described it and named it *Schistosomum turkestanicum* Skrjabin, 1913.

N.P. Popov (1926) found five specimens of this trematode in the veins of the liver of the cat (*Felis catus* dom.), on Muynak Island in the Aral Sea. The discovered trematodes were males that contained no females in the gynecophoral canal. L.G. Panova (1927, 1940) found schistosoma in the cattle of Kzyl Orda. The author inspected 205 livers, in 61 (30.3%) of which she found the parasites. Z.V. Wolf (1936) reports about the trematodes found *Sch. turkestanicum* in Kazakhstan. Boyev (1939, 1944, 1963) made research into helminths of the animals of Kazakhstan and noted that schistosomiasis was widely spread in the country, playing an important part in the animals' pathology. E.I. Pryadko (1962) reported about *Sch. Turkestanicum* in the cattle of the southeastern part of Kazakhstan.

In the 1960s, researchers carried out more detailed studies of schistosomiasis.

L.I. Lavrov (1963, 1964, 1966) wrote that *Sch. turkestanicum* are distributed only in the southern part of the northern hemisphere (below the 50th parallel) and that even there they concentrate only in some areas. This parasite was recorded mainly in animals living near immobile bodies of water or those with slow currents, that is, in the habitats of molluscs, their intermediate hosts. Further, the researcher reported that this trematode was the most common for the flood plain of the lower course of the Syrdarya River, where the rate of infection in cattle was 26%. In the middle course of the Syrdarya and in the Arys, the former's tributary, this trematode was much less common—2.1%. Schistosoma could be found in cattle in all seasons, with the highest infection rate in spring—28.3% in young animals and 30.8% in adult ones. The average rate of infection with this trematode is almost the same in young animals (26%) and in adults (25.3%); however, the number of parasite specimens found in young animals (45–660) is somewhat larger than that in adults (25–237).

L.I. Lavrov, V.Ya. Panin and K.K. Uvaliyeva (1974) note that schistosomiasis is mainly concentrated near the water bodies in the flood plain of the lower course of the Syrdarya River. There the rate of infection in cattle is 40%, reaching 68–70% at some farms.

In Kazakhstan, schistosomiasis animals are most common for the Syrdarya valley, for its lower course, where the infection rate in cattle is 26.0%, the flood plain of the middle course of the river features a much lesser portion of infected animals—2.1%, while the deserts and mountains of the country remain uninhabited by the parasites [4].

Based on the literary data on schistosomiasis of animals in Kazakhstan, we consider that the schistosomiasis situation in the areas in the middle and lower courses of the Syrdarya River is unstable. There high infection rates were recorded in synanthropic animals.

Azerbaijan. G.V. Kasimov (1942), S.M. Tuayev (1946) and N.M. Kolesnikov (1953) carried out research into schistosomiasis of the animals of the natural and synanthropic biocoenoses in Azerbaijan. According to Tuayev (1946), the trematode causing schistosomiasis (*Sch. turkestanicum*) was found in the zebu of Azerbaijan and Iran. The author inspected 23 zebu specimens (10 of which were from Iran) and 2 buffalos. Neither of the two dissected buffaloes had any traces of *Sch. turkestanicum*. As for the zebu, 7 of the dissected animals turned out to be infected with this trematode. The number of trematode specimens found in the Iranian zebu ranged between 1 and 14, and that in the Azerbaijani ones between 2 and 7838. The trematodes were detected in the vessels of the mesentery, under the mucous membrane of the small and large intestine, in the liver, lungs and spleen.

Synanthropic animals infected with schistosoma predominate over the wild ones in the countries of the former USSR. However, some areas of Uzbekistan and Russia are characterised by large numbers of wild animals infected with this trematode. It means that the natural and synanthropic biocoenoses are connected closely in terms of the distribution of schistosomiasis.

The materials on the distribution of schistosomiasis of animals in the countries of the former USSR indicate that the schistosomiasis situation is not stable, particularly in the areas where pasturing is one of the elements of cattle breeding. Currently, the tendency is seen towards a wide distribution of the infection in a number of Central Asian regions.

As we have a general picture of the distribution of the disease in the countries of the former USSR, we thought it expedient to analyse the problem in other countries around the world as well. We have enough literary data for it covering the period between 1908 and 2017. We also used our personal correspondence with foreign researchers.

Mongolia. Ye.Ye. Shumakovich (1936) recorded *Sch. turkestanicum* in the cattle and dzo of Mongolia. The researcher wrote: '...The part of the body this parasite concentrates in – the blood vessels of the liver – makes me think that a lodger like this one cannot but damage the organism, the more so as its close relation parasitising humans is known to cause a serious disease in the latter named "schistosomiasis." However, the disease of cattle has not studied at all – either its history or its epizootology, prevention or treatment'. S. Yamagiva (1931) also reported about this schistosoma found in the domestic animals of Mongolia.

China. Hsü (1938) began research into schistosomiasis of the synanthropic biocoenosis in the late 1930s. He recorded a rapid distribution of *Sch. turkestanicum* among sheep and goats in Zhejiang, Gansu, Jiangxi, Zhejiang and Hubei Provinces. The author also reported on cercarioses in humans caused by *Schistosoma* cercariae in the wetlands of China, where schistosomiasis is quite common.

Kuo (quoted from K. I. Skrjabin, 1951) recorded schistosomiasis in cattle in one of China's provinces, where the infection rate was 40.0%.

Z. Liu et al. (1987), Ch. Tang et al. (1983) and C. Wang et al. (2000, 2002, 2009) report about a wide distribution of *Sch. turkestanicum* among domestic animals and about cercarioses of humans caused by cercariae of this trematode in China.

Iraq. C. MacHattie (1936) made comprehensive research into schistosomiasis of animals in various regions of Iraq. The author indicated that the rate of infection with schistosoma in the sheep, goats, cattle and buffalos of the wetlands of the Tigris River was equal to 80.0%, while that in the horses, donkeys, mules and camels—about 15.0%.

Iran. In this country *Sch. turkestanicum* is widely distributed among synanthropic and wild animals. Since 1965 scientists have carried out a number of research works in the territory (F. Arfaa, H. Sabaghian, H. Ale-Bawood, 1965).

J. Massoud (1973, 1974), J. Massoud and G. Nelson (1973) also carried out a significant amount of research into schistosomiasis of domestic animals. They established the infection rate in cattle—30%, sheep—16%, goats—7% and buffalos—2%. Other researchers also report about schistosomiasis of animals and cercarioses of humans (Sahba, Malek, 1979; Athari et al., 1990, 2006; Farhnak, Essalat, 2003).

India. The research into the distribution of *Sch. turkestanicum* begun in the late 1950s and covered various regions of the country (H. Srivastava & K. Trisul (1957), S. Dutt & H. Srivastava (1964), V. Kumar (1973), F. Chauhan et al., (1973)). The schistosomiasis caused by this trematode species is distributed among cattle, buffalos, sheep, goats, horses, donkeys, mules and camels.

Pakistan. Schistosomiasis was recorded by M. Abdussalam and M. Sarvar (1953). S. Yasin (1959) reported that parasitic diseases were the main cause of the material losses suffered by the cattle breeding industry of Pakistan. He referred *Sch. turkestanicum* to pathogenic trematode species causing schistosomiasis.

France. We know about the distribution of *Sch. turkestanicum* in domestic animals from a personal oral message given by Doctor Euzeby from Lion (1973, personal message).

Turkey. For a long time, there had been only one report on *Sch. turkestanicum* in rats living in the wild [5]. Later Guralp, Finar (1982) confirmed the distribution of *Sch. turkestanicum* in sheep in the territory of Turkey.

Hungary. According to G. Majoros et al. (2010), *Sch. turkestanicum* was recorded in the European red deer (*Cervus elaphus*). Molluscs *L. auricularia* were reported to be the trematode's intermediate host. The researcher also noted the role of this trematode in the distribution of cercarioses in humans.

In the end of the survey on the distribution of schistosomiasis among synanthropic animals in different countries of the world, we should mention the message made by Doctor Vittoz (1959). He referred schistosomiasis (*Sch. turkestanicum*) to the main diseases of the zebu and buffalos in a number of Asian countries (India, Sri Lanka, Pakistan, Burma, Thailand, Laos, Cambodia, Vietnam and Indonesia).

The numerous materials on the distribution of schistosomiasis among synanthropic and wild animals in different countries of the world indicate that the infection causes great damage to their economies. It is evident that this problem resulted in the increase of the number of publications on this infection in animals in a number of Asian and European countries.

The results of our own research and the literary data [6–9] allow us to refer schistosomiasis (*Sch. turkestanicum*) to the feral nidal infections in all of its areas of distribution. The parasites causing the disease circulate in the wild regardless of the presence of wild animals in the area. They anyway cover the full cycle of their development and create nidi of infection in natural biocoenoses. In this case, schistosoma circulate in the natural biocoenoses, where wild animals (molluscs and wild vertebrates) act as their intermediate and definitive hosts, which is confirmed by Ya.N. Zakhryalov (1975). Thus, a natural nidus is a place where domestic animals become infected with schistosomiasis. In the mixed feral and synanthropic nidus of the infection the molluscs (wild animals) act as intermediate hosts and domestic animals—as definitive hosts.

Preconditions for the emergence of schistosomiasis caused by *Sch. turkestanicum* in the areas of the development, exploitation and irrigation of lands. Land reclamation occupies an important place in the present-day agrarian policy. In our days, it has become one of the priority tasks for the government.

Many of the country's regions are involved in the reclamation programme. Vast territories of Uzbekistan are being actively developed and irrigated.

We know that the construction of new irrigation systems leads to the formation of new bodies of water. The biocoenoses of these bodies of water are characterised by rich invertebrate fauna, which includes freshwater molluscs—trematodes intermediate hosts. Therefore, it is highly important to foresee possibilities for the formation of new concentrations of parasitic infections, including schistosomiasis, which may be caused by the implementation of the new reclamation programme.

The systematic research into the problem was divided into stages. The first stage aimed at the determination of the species composition of the molluscs inhabiting the bodies of water in the Republic of Karakalpakstan and Khorezm Province. The scientists also studied the molluscs' population density and the rate of infection with *Schistosoma turkestanicum* parthenitae and cercariae in the natural and artificial water bodies of the abovementioned regions with the unstable schistosomiasis situation. In addition, the researchers inspected domestic and wild animals to establish the rate of infection with populations of maritae of this trematode [2, 10, 11]. There the scientists recorded large numbers of molluscs *L. auricularia* and high rates of infection with schistosoma cercariae among them [12–16].

At the second stage, the research was carried out following a similar scheme, but this time in an area with a stable schistosomiasis situation, that is, in the south of Uzbekistan. The scientists inspected 5000 specimens of molluscs from different types of water bodies frequented by animals. They did not find any *Sch. turkestanicum* cercariae in molluscs, including the common species *L. auricularia*. No schistosoma were detected in hoofed animals either. It should be noted that both the biotic and abitoic conditions of the region are perfectly suitable for the emergence of the infection nidi, but the territory remains uninhabited by the parasite. This region currently features a stable schistosomiasis situation.

The main task of the third stage was to study the possibilities for the emergence of schistosomiasis in the areas, where the lands were to be developed and irrigated. The work was carried out in the northeastern part of Uzbekistan (Syrdarya, Jizzakh and Tashkent Provinces)—the area where the lands of the Golodnaya and Jizzakh steppes were being actively reclaimed. Prior to the reclamation, before the land was irrigated, no *Schistosoma* were found in the region. As the scientists were inspecting bodies of water and irrigation systems in the reclamation areas of Jizzakh and Syrdarya Provinces fed by the Syrdarya River, they recorded molluscs *L. auricularia*. The population density was rather high—up to 105 specimens per 1 m^2. The rate of infection with *Sch. turkestanicum* larvae in molluscs ranged between 0.3 and 0.6% [17]. Further research gave much higher figures—0.4-1.7%. In the course of the inspection of sheep and cattle, the researchers also recorded trematodes *Sch. turkestanicum* [1, 14, 15, 18].

The large-scale reclamation of the lands of the Golodnaya and Jizzakh steps created rapidly all biological preconditions necessary for the natural circulation of this schistosoma in this region of Uzbekistan. We suppose that the infection was brought by the definitive hosts, while the favourable environment, in particular, the bodies of water and temperatures, created new infection nidi. The distributive role of the molluscs, the trematodes' intermediate hosts that came to this area with the water of the irrigation canals, should also be taken into consideration. It is important, as the areas of both the middle and the lower courses of the Syrdarya are not stable in terms of schistosomiasis [19]. Here, we can observe the expansion of the range of this trematode caused by the human impact on the environment.

Turkmenistan faces a similar situation. The construction of the Karakum canal and the conveyance of water from the Amudarya across the Karakum desert to the southern and southwestern regions of the country contributed to the creation of favourable conditions in that area for freshwater molluscs (*L. auricularia*), schistosoma intermediate hosts, and led to schistosomiasis in sheep and cattle.

Thus, the information given above demonstrates that new schistosomiasis nidi in certain regions of Central Asia, including the areas where the land is developed and irrigated, may form if proper conditions for the development of the trematode are created in these regions [10, 17]. The large-scale reclamation of lands has rapidly created a tendency to a vast distribution of schistosomiasis.

In this connection, we should like to discuss some factors that contribute to the distribution of the infection in the mentioned regions.

In our opinion, this is connected with the nearness of the developed and irrigated lands to the regions with unstable schistosomiasis situations and the use of the waters of the Amudarya and Syrdarya for the reclamation, as vast portions of their basins lie in stationarily unstable areas in terms of schistosomiasis. This factor makes it possible for infected animals and parasitised molluscs *L. auricularia* to come to the reclaimed areas from the unstable territories. The situation is aggravated by the traditional trade in livestock among the people of various regions of Central Asia. In the last case, the distance factor is not significant at all.

The definitive host carries the infection from the unstable areas to the stable territories that are being reclaimed and irrigated, and thus the 'links of the epizootologic chain (the parasite—the intermediate host—the definitive host) connect' [20]. All this is possible under favourable temperature conditions. The materials of this section prove that schistosoma of our region like warm areas with an effective temperature of 5000–6100 degrees. This is enough for a five- or sixfold parthenogenesis in the intermediate host (a total of about 725–750^{0}C of an effective temperature is required for one parthenogenesis generation). The number of sunny hours in the region is between 2500 and 3059. The areas with schistosoma feature a solar radiation of 140–160 kcal per 1 cm^2 throughout a year. Schistosoma are not recorded in regions where the total radiation is below 130 kcal.

The geographical coincidence of the maximal solar radiation with *Sch. turkestanicum*'s habitats indicates the specificity of this trematode—its love for warmth. Therefore, the habitat of the species is conditioned, first of all, by climate. In this respect, all the territories of Central Asia (except for mountains and deserts) can become a potential habitat for schistosoma, as large-scale irrigation programmes are implemented. Schistosomiasis nidi can form in the Transcaucasian countries, and particularly in Azerbaijan, as it is situated close to Turkey and Iran—countries with an unstable schistosomiasis situation.

Therefore, to prevent the development of the disease it is necessary to exclude its penetration with the definitive hosts from unstable regions to reclamation areas. To do it, it is necessary to develop and follow strictly quarantine measures, which would be connected with the introduction of the animals into the farms of various types, and to follow strict regulations concerning various operations with livestock at private farms.

It is the first time that the impact of reclamation, development and irrigation on the distribution of schistosomiasis is estimated in this section, which conforms with the opinions of various researchers [21–23], who forecast the spacious distribution of other species of trematodes in other objects. Our research allowed us to forecast the possibility of emergence and development of new schistosomiasis nidi in Uzbekistan and Turkmenistan [17]. The forecast has been confirmed by the situation in the irriated areas of Uzbekistan and Turkmenistan [9, 24].

Author details

Djalaliddin A. Azimov[1], Bakhrom T. Norkobilov[2], Firuza D. Akramova[1] and Ulugbek A. Shakarbaev[1]

1 Institute of Zoology of the Academy of Sciences of the Republic of Uzbekistan, Tashkent, Uzbekistan

2 State Committee of Veterinary and Livestock Development of The Republic of Uzbekistan, Tashkent, Uzbekistan

*Address all correspondence to: afarov-alisher@mail.ru

References

[1] Azimov DA, Sultanov MA, Dadayev S. On helminths of the domestic animals of Jizzakh Province. The Uzbek Biological Magazine. Tashkent: Fan; 1979;**6**:54-57

[2] Azimov DA. To the Study of Orientobilharziasis in the Sheep, Goats and Cattle of Uzbekistan//the Materials of a Scientific Conference. 2. Moscow; 1965. pp. 8-9

[3] Azimov D.A. The New in Orientobilharziasis Control. The Agriculture of Uzbekistan//the Uzbek Biological Journal. Tashkent: Fan; 1977;**10**:51-53

[4] Lavrov LI. Materias on Orientobilharziasis in Kazakhstan. The Materials of a Scientific Conference.1. Moscow: Nauka; 1963;**1**:176

[5] Witenberg GC, Lengy J. A case of natural infection of field rats with *Ornithobilharzia turkestanica*. Refuah Veterinarith. 1966;23(1):64-67

[6] Boyev SN. The Significance of the Nidi Character of Helminthiases in the Helminthiasis Control. The Problems of Parasitology. Kiev; Наукова Думка, 1963. pp. 84-86

[7] Zakhryalov YN. Orientobilharziaturkestanica (Skrjabin, 1913) Dutt and Srivastava, 1955 in the Far East: The Abstract of a Doctoral Thesis. Alma-Ata; 1975. p. 43

[8] Majoros G, Dan A, Erdelyi K. A natural focus of the blood fluke *Orientobilharzia turkestanica* (Skrjabin, 1913) (Trematoda: Schistosomatidae) in red deer (*Cervus elaphus*) in Hungary. Veterinary Parasitology. 2010;**170**(3-4):218-223

[9] Azimov DA, Akramova FD, Shakarbayev UA, Shakarboyev EB. Orientobildgarsii - Mammalian Trematodes. Tashkent: Fan; 2014. p. 224

[10] Azimov DA. The biology of Ornithobilharzia turkestanica in Uzbekistan. Report by the Academy of Sciences. Tashkent: Fan; 1969;**7**:52-53

[11] Azimov DA. The restructuring of the trematode system of the suborder Schistosomatata Skrjabin et Schulz, 1937. The Zoological Magazine. 1970;**69**(8):1126-1131

[12] Azimov DA, Nurmukhamedov KN. Orientobilharziasis in ruminants. Journal agriculture of Uzbekistan. Mekhnat, Tashkent. 1967;**7**:56-58

[13] Azimov DA, Nurmukhamedov KN. New data on the biology of trematode Orientobilharzia turkestanica (Schistosomatidae). The Zoological Journal. 1968;**10**:1471-1478

[14] Shakarboyev EB. The Ecological and Functional Interrelations of Orientobilharzia Turkestanica (Skrjabin, 1913) – Bos taurus Linnaeus, 1758 in the Parasite-Host System: A PhD Thesis in Biology. Tashkent: Institute of Zoology. 1996. p. 134

[15] Shakarboyev EB. Trematodes of the Vertebrates of Uzbekistan (the Species Composition, Circulation Ways, Ecology Ad Biology): A Doctoral Thesis in Biology. Tashkent: Institute of Zoology. 2009. p. 243

[16] Kojabayev M. The Associative Infection with Trematodes in the Cattle (Bos taurus, Linnaeus, 1758) of the Aral Sea Area: A PhD Thesis. Tashkent: Institute of Zoology. 2001. p. 98

[17] Azimov DA. On the habitats of trematodes from the genus Orientobilharzia. The Uzbek Biological Journal. Tashkent: Fan; 1978;**3**:44-46

[18] Matchanov NM, Dadayev S. The zoogeographical characteristics of the helminthic fauna in the ungulates of Uzbekistan. The Uzbek Biological Journal. Tashkent: Fan; 1981;**4**:57-60

[19] Lavrov LI. The Rate of Infection with Ornithobilharzia in the Cattle of South Kazakhstan//Parasites of the Agricultural Animals of. 3. Kazakhstan: Alma-Ata; 1964. pp. 108-113

[20] Matekin PV, Shalayeva NM. Some patterns of distribution of agricultural animals' helminthiases in forest-steppe landscapes (for the understanding of the epizootological chain). The Zoological Journal. Moscow: Nauka; 1964;7:965-974

[21] Mereminsky AI. Paramphistomatoses of Cattle in Ukrainian Polesia (the Study of Epizootology, Forecast, Diagnostics, Therapy and Prevention): The Abstract of a Doctoral Thesis in Veterinary Sciences. Moscow: All-Union Institute of Helminthology named after K.I. Scriabin. 1971. p. 41

[22] Aleksandrov MV. The Heat of the Atmosphere and the Poikilothermal Aerobes Development Forecast. Tashkent: Fan; 1974. p. 164

[23] Sazanov AM. The Biological Principles of Prevention of Fascioliasis on Irrigated or Drained Lands: The Abstract of a Doctoral Thesis in Biology. Moscow: Всесоюзный институт гельминтологии имени К.И. Скрябина. 1976. p. 43

[24] Azimov DA, Akramova FD, Shakarboyev EB, Norqobilov BT, Shakarbayev UA, Sayitqulov BS. Schistosomiasis of Animals. Tashkent: Fan; 2019. p. 320

Chapter 7

The Clinical Course and Diagnosis of Schistosomiasis of Animals

Djalaliddin A. Azimov, Bakhrom T. Norkobilov, Alisher A. Safarov and Firuza D. Akramova

Abstract

The clinical manifestations of experimental schistosomiasis in animals are diverse, and the state of several stages is as follows: the first stage of the disease is characterised by cercariasis, dermatitis, general hyperaemia, increased body temperature, increased heart rate and respiration are observed. These changes are typical for the first 10–12 days after infection of animals; the second stage is characterised by the absence of noticeable violations of the physiological functions of the body, which coincides in time with the growth period and development of schistosomes in the blood vessels of the animal; the third (acute) stage of the disease manifests itself 5–6 weeks after infection of the animals and is characterised by progressive diarrhoea mixed with blood and fibrinous films. The coat is dishevelled, and the animal is emaciated. Puffiness is noted. With such symptoms, heavily infected animals die. The intensity of the invasion reaches 950 thousand ind. in individual animals. An acute course of schistosomiasis in cattle was observed in September–October 1964–1965, 1984–1985, 2004–2005 in the Republic of Karakalpakstan and Khorezm region. Only for the period 1984–1985 in the Republic of Karakalpakstan, more than 13 thousand heads of cattle died due to schistosomiasis caused by *Sch. turkestanicum*. An intravital diagnosis is based on the detection of eggs in animal faeces. Post-mortem diagnosis is made by examining the blood vessels of the liver and intestines, that is, method of complete helminthological dissections.

Keywords: schistosomiasis, *Sch. turkestanicum*, clinical course, stage, ovoscopy, autopsy

1. Introduction

The issues of the clinical presentations and diagnosis of schistosomiasis (*Sch. turkestanicum*), as well as the immunity against this disease, have been studied by a number of researchers and generalised by Azimov et al. 2014, 2019.

2. The clinical course of schistosomiasis of animals

According to our observations, the clinical presentations of schistosomiasis are diverse and correspond with those structural, functional and biochemical changes in the organism that form the set of the signs of this disease pathogenesis.

Experimenting on cattle infected with schistosomiasis we distinguished several phases.

The *first stage* of the disease is characterised by dermatitis, total hyperaemia, fever and rapid pulse and breathing. These pathological changes are characteristics of for the first 10–12 days after infection.

The *second stage* is characterised by the absence of any noticeable malfunctions in the organism, which coincides in time with the growth and development of schistosoma in the blood vessels of the animal.

The *third (acute) stage* comes 5–6 weeks after the infection and is characterised by progressing diarrhoea, and the faeces mixed with blood and pseudomembranes. All the clinical presentations are the clearest at this stage: the pale conjunctiva, fever with a temperature rising to 41.6°C, the pulse rate up to 180, arrhythmia and rapid breathing up to 120 inhalations and exhalations per minute. The hair is ruffled, and the animal looks oedematic and exhausted. At this time, an animal infected with a large number of parasites may die.

Ya.N. Zakhryalov (1975) observed calves infected experimentally with cercariae. He recorded dermatitis, total hyperaemia, oedema, fever, painfulness, spotted and striped haemorrhages along the veins (after the animal had died and been dissected). These changes can be seen within the first two or three days and disappear by the 10th day. During the whole period of the disease, the researcher recorded decrease in the number of erythrocytes and haemoglobin and an increase in sugar in the blood, leucocytes and globulin; the malfunction of the liver and considerable decrease of the liver weight, which is confirmed by our research [1].

The acute presentations of schistosomiasis in cattle were recorded in 1964–1965, 1984–1985 and 2004–2005 in the Republic of Karakalpakstan and Khorezm Province. In the period between 1984 and 1985, 13 thousand specimens of cattle died of diseases caused by trematodes, mainly of schistosomiasis, in the Republic of Karakalpakstan [1, 2]. The diseased animals were strongly exhausted, their breathing was too rapid, the visible parts of their mucous membranes were pale, while the hair was ruffled. The animals also suffered from diarrhoea, and their faeces were mixed with blood and fibrinogenous membranes.

The strong diarrhoea makes the animals stand permanently in a defecation pose. The animals with such symptoms die in two or three days. Hundreds of thousands of parasites were discovered in the blood vessels of the dissected animals after they died, while their organs had the characteristic of pathological changes.

Having analysed the material, we could make quite a clear picture of the disease's clinical course in animals, which is highly valuable for the timely diagnosis of the infection.

3. The diagnosis of schistosomiasis in animals

To diagnose the disease while the animal is still alive, the following methods are used: the successive faeces washing method; the miracidoscopy method; the allergic and antibody-mediated methods [3–12].

To check the reliability of the methods used in the detection of miracidia that have just gone out of the schistosom eggs, we used the faeces of infected animals.

The most effective methods for lifetime diagnostics of schistosomiasis in animals are the methods of precipitation of eggs and miracidioscopy.

The *successive washing method* is based on the precipitation of the eggs of this trematode. To do it, you should take 5–10 g of faeces, place them in a glass and add water; the ratio of the water to the faeces must be 10:1. Filter the substance through a sieve or gauze. Then fill the glass with water. Keep the substance undisturbed for 5–10 minutes and pour out the upper layer of the fluid. Then again add water to the remaining substance. You should wash the substance several times, until the poured fluid is transparent. Then place the sediment on a microscope slide or in a Petri dish using a pipette. It is advisable that you use cold water (10–15°C) for this procedure, as at higher temperatures the eggs would emit *Sch. turkestanicum* miracidia.

The research showed that this method was quite effective for the lifetime diagnostics of schistosomiasis in animals of 85–100%.

The *miracidioscopy method* is based on the extraction of miracidia from the faeces of infected animals, which is described in Chapter 2.

4. Posthumous diagnostics of schistosomiasis in animals

Veins, and particularly those in the mesentery and liver, are *Schistosoma*'s favourite places of parasitising. It would be enough to watch a loop of the intestine with blood vessels at high illuminations in order to see a large number of milky-white trematodes in the veins.

To diagnose accurately and properly you should inspect the animals using the method of total helminthological dissection developed by K.I. Skrjabin (1928), with the dissection of blood vessels.

Author details

Djalaliddin A. Azimov[1], Bakhrom T. Norkobilov[2], Alisher A. Safarov[2]* and Firuza D. Akramova[1]

1 Institute of Zoology of the Academy of Sciences of the Republic of Uzbekistan, Tashkent, Uzbekistan

2 State Committee of Veterinary and Livestock Development of the Republic of Uzbekistan, Tashkent, Uzbekistan

*Address all correspondence to: safarov-alisher@mail.ru

References

[1] Azimov DA. Tremadodes—Parasites of Animals and Human. Tashkent: Mehnat; 1986. p. 128

[2] Shakiyev YS, Oripov AO. The phenomenon of accumulation of trematodes in the wild of the southern part of the Aral Sea area. In: The Scientific Provision of Veterinary Stability in the Cattle Breeding of Uzbekistan. The Thesis of the Report of the Scientific Conference Dedicated to the 70th Anniversary. Samarkand: Uzbek Veterinary research Institute; 1996. pp. 182-185

[3] Zakhryalov YN. On the effectiveness of the ovoscopic and larvoscopic methods of diagnosing orientobilharziasis caused by Ornithobilharzia turkestanica in cattle. The Materials of a Scientific Conference. Moscow. 1966;**Part 1**:111-116

[4] Zakhryalov YN. To the question of the peroral way of infecting with *Ornithobilharzia turkestanica*. In: The Materials of the Scientific Conference. Blagoveshchensk; 1971. pp. 67-69

[5] Zakhryalov YN. Orientobilharziaturkestanica (Skrjabin, 1913) Dutt and Srivastava, 1955 in the Far East: The abstract of a doctoral thesis. Alma-Ata: Institute of Zoology; 1975. p. 43

[6] Azimov DA. The issues of the epizootology of orientobilharziasis in ruminants. Veterinariya. 1966;**11**:50-52

[7] Azimov DA. The biology of Ornithobilharzia turkestanica in Uzbekistan. Report by the Academy of Sciences. 1969;7:52-53

[8] Azimov DA. On the habitats of trematodes from the genus Orientobilharzia. The Uzbek Biological Journal. Tashkent: Fan; 1978;**3**:44-46

[9] Stepanov DF. Ornitobilharziosis of animals in Turkmen SSR and the experimental therapy of this helminthiasis: The abstract of a PhD thesis in the veterinary science. M., 1969. p. 18

[10] Massoud J. Studies on the Schistosomes of domestic animals in Iran. I. Observations on Ornithobilharzia turkestanica (Skrjabin, 1913) in Khuzestan. Journal of Helminthology. 1973;**67**(2):165-180

[11] Shakarboyev EB. The structure of the trematode fauna in the mammals of Uzbekistan. In: The Bulletin of the Karakalpaki Department of the Academy of Sciences of the Republic of Uzbekistan. Vol. 3. Nukus: Academy of Sciences; 2008. pp. 25-27

[12] Azimov DA, Akramova FD, Shakarbayev UA, Shakarboyev EB. Orientobildgarsii—Mammalian Trematodes. Tashkent: Fan; 2014. p. 224

Chapter 8

The Treatment and Prevention of Schistosomiasis of Animals

Djalaliddin A. Azimov, Bakhrom T. Norkobilov, Firuza D. Akramova, Ulugbek A. Shakarbaev and Alisher A. Safarov

Abstract

The chapter is devoted to finding methods and means of deworming animals. Of the tested drugs—Ambilgar, Antimosan, Miracil D, Praziquantel and Droncit (praziquantel) turned out to be the most effective. The anthelmintic efficacy of Ambilgar at a dose of 20–25 mg/kg of live weight in sheep, goats and cattle ranged from 85 to 100%. Praziquantel, administered orally at a dose of 20–25 mg/kg of sheep and cattle weight, proved to be a highly effective anthelmintic against schistosomiasis in animals, where the extensive effectiveness was up to 100%. Currently, this drug is widely used for the treatment and prevention of animal schistosomiasis in the farms of Uzbekistan.

Keywords: schistosomiasis, sheep, goat, cattle, deworming, anthelmintic, ambilgar, droncit, praziquantel, miracil, antimosan

1. Introduction

In the course of the research, we studied the biology of the parasite and the epizootology of schistosomiasis in animals. There are several vulnerable links in the chain of the infection circulation; by breaking these links we shall achieve the best preventive effect. The methods are to break the endogenous phase in the development of the parasite in the organism of the definitive host and to prevent the contact of the miracidia with the molluscs and the cercariae with the vertebrates. We must have an integrated approach, using different methods and means, to break the chain.

2. Exploring the methods and means of dehelminthisation of animals

Studying different questions concerning the control of schistosomiasis, we obtained interesting data on the treatment of animals infected with *Sch. turkestanicum* [1].

At the first stage, we tested a number of medicinal agents on animals infected with schistosomiasis naturally or experimentally. The medicines included Ambilgar, Antimosan and Miracil D. The most effective was Ambilgar.

Ambilgar (CIBA-32644-Ba, Niridazole, Nitroimidazole) is the chemical 1-(5-nitro-2-thiazole)-2-imidazole (niridazole). This is a conservative substance, which is yellowish, tasteless and poorly soluble in water. It is produced in the form of tablets. The medicine is highly effective against schistosomiasis in human and animals [2–6].

We tested Ambilgar on 40 rabbits, 30 sheep, 30 goats and 23 calves infected with *Sch. turkestanicum,* comparing the results with a reference group.

We gave Ambilgar to the experimental animals per orally, in doses of 15, 20 and 30 mg/kg, two and three times with an interval of 5 days. In 12–15 days after the last dose, we dissected the animals. As we dissected the rabbits from the experimental and reference groups, we established the following fact: the extenseffectiveness was 80.0% in the 15 mg/kg dose (three times), while its inteseffectiveness was 84.0%; about 20 and 30 mg/kg doses (two times) gave a 100.0% extenseffectiveness and inteseffectiveness. Almost the same results were obtained as we had tested ambilgar on sheep, goats, and calves, in doses of 15, 20 and 30 mg per 1 kg of liver weight. We established that the antihelminthic effectiveness of ambilgar as an anti-schistosomiasis agent was 85.0–100.0%.

Therefore, we established that to treat schistosomiasis the optimal dosage of this medicine was 20 mg/kg for rabbits, 20–25 mg/kg for sheep and goats and 30–40 mg/kg for calves, respectively.

The animals did not show any obvious deviation from the norm either in the first days after the dehelminthisation or in the following days.

According to Krotov's biological classification (1973), Ambilgar belongs to medicines affecting the helminths' energetic processes. It suppresses glycolysis in mature blood flukes. The medicine accumulates mainly in the genital system and the eggs. The eggs stop developing. The break in the egg-laying process means that the trematodes' gonads are damaged. Ambilgar suppresses the activity of glucose 6-phosphate dehydrogenase in blood flukes. The researcher considers that the imidazole ring and its nitro group are the active principles blocking the enzymes.

Ambilgar is absorbed well from the gastrointestinal tract and disintegrates quickly in the liver. The disintegration products of this chemical are egested through the kidneys. In this case, the urine becomes orange, then brown and even black. In 24–36 hours, the colour of the urine becomes normal again [3].

Among the second-stage medicines we tested, the most effective against schistosomiasis were Droncit and Azinoks.

The medicinal agents were tested in 1984–1996 on a large population of cattle strongly infected with schistosoma, at the farms of Kegeyli and Kungrad Districts of the Republic of Karakalpakstan.

Droncit (Praziquantelum) 2-cyclohexilcarbonil-11, 3, 4, 6, 7, 11 v—hexahydro—24-pirazino 2.1—a – izochinoline. This medicine is manufactured by Bayer (Germany) as an antihelminthic agent used against cestodiases of dogs. It is in the form of tablets.

The pure medicine is colourless fine-grained crystalline powder, soluble in chloroform and spirit and hardly soluble in water. The melting temperature is 136–140°C slightly toxic. The LD_{50} for mice and rats is from 1000 to 7000 mg/kg.

Droncit was tested on 200 specimens of cattle of different age and sex with the purpose of development of the pattern and doses (**Table 1**).

In 15 days after the experimental and reference animals took Droncit (individually, per orally), we dissected them at the slaughterhouse of Nukus and inspected them. About 25 mg/kg dose of the medicine turned out to be effective for animals infected with schistosomiasis.

No.	Group of animals	Number of animals	Dose/q-ty of times	EE, %
1.	Experimental group	50	15 mg/kg, two times	60.0
2.	Experimental group	50	20 mg/kg, two times	80.0
3.	Experimental group	50	25 mg/kg, two times	100.0
4.	Reference group	50	No medicine was given	—

Table 1.
Droncit test pattern for cattle infected with schistosomiasis.

Azinoks is a Russia-made analogue of Droncit, synthetised at the Institute of Medical Parasitology and Tropical Medicine (Moscow). It is manufactured by the Usolye Sibirskoye Chemical and Pharmaceutical Plant under the Ministry of Health and Medical Industry and is intended to cure opisthorchiasis of humans.

The medicine has the form of white powder with the специфическим of smell. We carried out experiments at the farms of the Republic of Karakalpakstan to determine the doses of Azinoks. We used 108 specimens of cattle infected sporadically with *Sch. turkestanicum* for the experiments.

The experiments demonstrated that the 15 mg/kg dose of Azinoks gave little effect, 20 mg/kg was effective enough (EE–66.6%), while the doses of 25, 35 and 50 mg/kg were highly effective (EE–100%). The number of schistosoma specimens in experimental animals ranged between 45 and 175 thousand. After the animals took the medicine, they did not show any morphological or physiological changes.

Thus, 25 mg/kg of Azinoks is a therapeutic dose in the cure of schistosomiasis in cattle.

According to our research, Droncit (Praziquantelum) leads to various types of dystrophies of *Sch. turkestanicum*'s tissues and organs, as well as to irreversible degenerative changes in the males and females of the trematode.

The high effectiveness of Droncit (Praziquantelum) means that the medicine can be used widely to cure schistosomiasis of animals.

3. The principles of prevention of schistosomiasis in animals

For the full prevention of schistosomiasis, as we believe, an integrated approach is needed. One of the extremely important components of the complex of measures is the fight against mollusks - intermediate hosts in limited and intense foci of invasions.

In theory, there are three ways to control molluscs, the intermediate hosts of the studied trematode: biological control; destruction of the molluscs' biotopes by draining wetlands and swampy pastures and cleaning bodies of water; amelioration of pastures by destroying the molluscs with the help of molluscicides.

We tested blue stone and 5.4-dichlorsalicylanilid in prescribed concentrations as substances potentially effective against molluscs, *Schistosoma*'s intermediate hosts.

Blue stone water solutions of 1:5.000, 1:10,000 and 1:25.000 kill 100% of ear pond snails and, together with them, destroy 100% of *Schistosoma* larvae.

5.4-dichlorsalicylanilid solutions of 1:500.000 and 1:1.000.000 do the same, killing 100% of *Schistosoma* larvae and *Lymnaea auricularia*.

The anti-mollusc agents are splattered in the biotopes of the ear pond snails in the period, when they are most active. In Uzbekistan, this period is usually June, July and August.

The draining of wet-pasturing areas is also important for the prevention of schistosomiasis in animals.

It should be noted that it is highly important to transfer the animals onto the industry-based breeding for successful prevention of helminthiases, including schistosomiasis. The change in the animal keeping technology would break the contact between the parasite and the sensitive animal.

By now scientists have developed necessary prerequisites to decrease the rate of infection with schistosomiasis in animals and to liquidate infection in certain nidi. This is achieved through a complex of medical and preventive measures and through the use of progressive methods and cattle breeding technologies.

Thus, the strategy of schistosomiasis control must aim for a decrease in the transmission of the infection through decrease in the mollusc population; dehelminthisation of animals carrying the disease; the creation of new, more effective medicines; the improvement of the organisational structure of the anti-epizootic services; and strict accordance with the veterinary and sanitary norms at farms and in the wild [7–13].

The results of the complex research allowed us to develop and test entirely new methods and means of prevention of schistosomiasis:

- Replacement of the pastures unstable in terms of schistosomiasis from June to October (the most effective measure).

- Draining of wetlands, which makes the living conditions unfavourable for molluscs and leads to the decrease of their population. In this respect, subsurface drainage should be given special attention.

- Keeping of animals in stalls.

- Separation of young and adult animals and their grazing in areas stable in terms of schistosomiasis.

- Improvement of the sanitary conditions of water bodies and drinking places.

- Biothermal disinfection of dung.

- Particularly dangerous biotopes should be treated with anti-mollusc agents, such as blue stone, dissolved at a ratio of 1:5.000 and 5.4-dichlorsalicylanilid (1:500.000 and 1:1.000.000). These agents reduce mollusc populations and kill the parasite's larvae. The anti-mollusc agents should be used from May to September.

- Preventive dehelminthisation of cattle with the use of anti-helminthic agents, to which *Schistosoma* are sensitive, such as Droncit and Azinoks. The first series of preventive measures should be taken in May, the second one in September and the third series in December or January.

Author details

Djalaliddin A. Azimov[1], Bakhrom T. Norkobilov[2], Firuza D. Akramova[1], Ulugbek A. Shakarbaev[1] and Alisher A. Safarov[2]*

1 Institute of Zoology of the Academy of Sciences of the Republic of Uzbekistan, Tashkent, Uzbekistan

2 State Committee of Veterinary and Livestock Development of the Republic of Uzbekistan, Tashkent, Uzbekistan

*Address all correspondence to: safarov-alisher@mail.ru

References

[1] Azimov DA. The biology of trematode Trichobilharzia ocellata in Uzbekistan (Schistosomatata: Ornithobilharziidae). In: The Uzbek Biological Magazine. Vol. 3. Tashkent: Fan; 1977. pp. 44-46

[2] Krotov AI. The Principles of the Experimental Therapy of Helminthiases. Moscow: Meditsina; 1973. p. 272

[3] Zolotukhin SI. Textbook in Pharmacology. Moscow: Medicine; 1975. p. 296

[4] Jackson H, Davies P, Bock M. Chemosterilization of Schistosoma mansoni. Nature. 1968;**218**(5145):977

[5] Ahluwalia S. Chemotherapy of Schistosomisis incognitum in pig. 3. Ambilhar and miracil-D. Indian Journal of Animal Sciences. 1973;**5**:428-434

[6] Muraleedharan K, Kumar SP, Hegde KS, Alwar VS. Comparative efficacy of neguvon, ambilhar and sodium tartarate against nasal schistosomiasis in cattle. The Indian Veterinary Journal. 1977;**54**(9):703-708

[7] Azimov DA. Tremadodes—Parasites of Animals and Human. Tashkent: Mekhnat; 1986. p. 128

[8] Shakarboyev EB. The Ecological and Functional Interrelations of *Orientobilharzia Turkestanica* (Skrjabin, 1913)—Bos taurus Linnaeus, 1758 in the Parasite-Host System: A PhD Thesis in Biology. Tashkent: Institute of Zoology; 1996. p. 134

[9] Kojabayev M. The Associative Infection with Trematodes in the Cattle (Bos taurus, Linnaeus, 1758) of the Aral Sea Area: A PhD Thesis. Tashkent: Institute of Zoology; 2001. p. 98

[10] Shakarboev EB, Akramova FZ, Golovanov VI, Azimov DA. Recommendations for the Prevention of Schistosomatosis in Livestock and Poultry. Tashkent; 2008. p. 27

[11] Azimov DA, Shakarboyev EB, Akramova FD, Shakarbayev UA. Orientobilgartsioz: Diagnostika and profilaktika (handout). Tashkent; 2010. p. 8

[12] Azimov DA, Akramova FD, Shakarbayev UA, Shakarboyev EB. Orientobildgarsii—Mammalian Trematodes. Tashkent: Fan; 2014. p. 224

[13] Azimov DA, Akramova FD, Shakarboyev EB, Norqobilov BT, Shakarbayev UA, Sayitqulov BS. Schistosomiasis of Animals. Tashkent: Fan; 2019. p. 320

Chapter 9

Cercarioses of Humans Caused by Cercariae of *Schistosoma Turkestanicum* Skrjabin 1913

Firuza D. Akramova, Djalaliddin A. Azimov, Ulugbek A. Shakarbaev and Alisher A. Safarov

Abstract

This chapter is devoted to the problem of human cercariasis, parasitic diseases caused by cercariae (larvae) of trematodes of the family Schistosomatidae, parasitising in a mature (marita) state in the circulatory system of mammals and water birds. Man is not a specific host for them, however, schistosomatid cercariae, including *Schistosoma turkestanicum*, are able to actively penetrate through its skin in a pond, causing skin lesions (dermatitis) and toxic effects. It pays great attention to the spread of human cercariasis and clinical manifestations of the disease in Uzbekistan and other countries of Asia and Europe. Examples of the spread of cercariasis and their foci in the reservoirs of the Amudarya, Syrdarya, Chirchik rivers within Uzbekistan and their prevention will be seen.

Keywords: cercarial dermatitis, cercariasis, nonspecific host, foci, reservoirs, prevention

1. Cercarioses of Humans Caused by Cercariae of *Schistosoma Turkestanicum* Skrjabin 1913

Cercarioses are parasitic diseases caused by cercariae of trematodes from the order Schistosomatidae, the mature forms of which parasitise in the blood system of warm-blooded animals—aquatic and semi-aquatic birds and mammals.

The human is a non-specific host for trematode species from the families Bilharziellidae and Schistosomatidae. In the course of numerous studies, researchers established that cercariae of Bilharziellidae and Schistosomatidae are able to penetrate through the skin of humans when contacting them in bodies of water containing larvae produced by infected molluscs from the families Lymnaeidae, Planorbidae, Bulynidae, Physidae and Melanoididae. Cercarioses may be caught while bathing, playing in water, washing clothes, carrying out agricultural, reclamation, research or other work in water or walking bare-footed on wet grass near swampy bodies of water (Bear, Voronin, 2007).

The main strategy used by cercariae of the studied trematode to infect specific and non-specific hosts is to stick to the host's skin and actively penetrate through it inside the organism. Penetrating through the host's skin cercariae cause numerous mechanical injuries to the skin, on the one hand, and, on the other hand, intoxicate the host's organism with their metabolic and decay products, sensibilise it with cercariae antigen and weaken the immune system [1–9].

Cercariae of Schistosomatidae have long since been known to attack humans and cause cercarioses; however, it became a medical and biological problem of urban ecosystems only a few decades ago, which was rightly pointed out by Bear, Voronin (2007).

According to modern concepts, active nidi of human cercarioses caused by cercariae *Sch. turkestanicum* are recorded in a number of countries throughout Asia and Europe [10–24].

Cercariae of this schistosoma are able to penetrate through the skin when contacting it in bodies of water containing infected freshwater molluscs from the genus *Lymnaea* (=*Radix*).

It should be noted that cercariae of *Sch. turkestanicum*that have penetrated the organism of the definitive host (mammal) cause the first stage of diseases named cercarioses. This results from the penetration of the cercariae through the skin and the migration of schistosomules in the host's organism. It was established that the schistosome species parasitising humans in endemic nidi also cause the first stage of cercariosis.

Therefore, blood flukes cause cercarioses in both the specific and non-specific hosts of the studied schistosoma.

Which territories (reservoirs, their separate zones) can be considered microfoci of cercariasis, and which ones can not, depends on the situation in them with lung mollusks that act as intermediate hosts of schistosomes: their presence in water bodies, population density, susceptibility to invasion, invasion by parthenites schistosomes in specific water bodies and, finally, on the density of schistosome cercariae in individual water bodies and their zones.

For many years, carrying out scientific research into schistosomiasis in the Aral Sea area, we were informed by local people about specific bites and red spots on their legs they suffered when collecting rush to feed the cattle in water and when working in a rice field. We have often observed cercarioses in our fellow-researchers who worked in water collecting molluscs *Lymnaea*, *Sch. turkestanicum* hosts in areas with cercarioses nidi (**Figures 1** and **2**).

Let us describe the character of cercarioses caused by cercariae *Sch. turkestanicum* in Uzbekistan.

Cercarioses are characterised by bites and red spots on the legs—only in the parts that have been underwater. After the person leaves the water, they feel slight prickling on the skin, which turns rather bright red. It is enough to stay for 10–15 minutes in such water to feel strongly these symptoms. Hardly bearable pruritus is one of the presentations of the disease. The pruritus appears 1–2, sometimes 5–6 hours later, gradually intensifying, particularly in the nighttime.

If the number of cercariae penetrating the skin is great, the itch becomes so strong that the infected person cannot sleep and work properly. By the end of the day, the person feels slightly feverous, indisposed, asthenic and agitated; they cough and feel pain in the chest.

In the following days the itching continues, rash appearing in the itching places in the form of small reddish mounds the size of a millet grain (see the coloured insert, **Figure 3**). Sometime later red papules appear, on the top of which blisters filled with

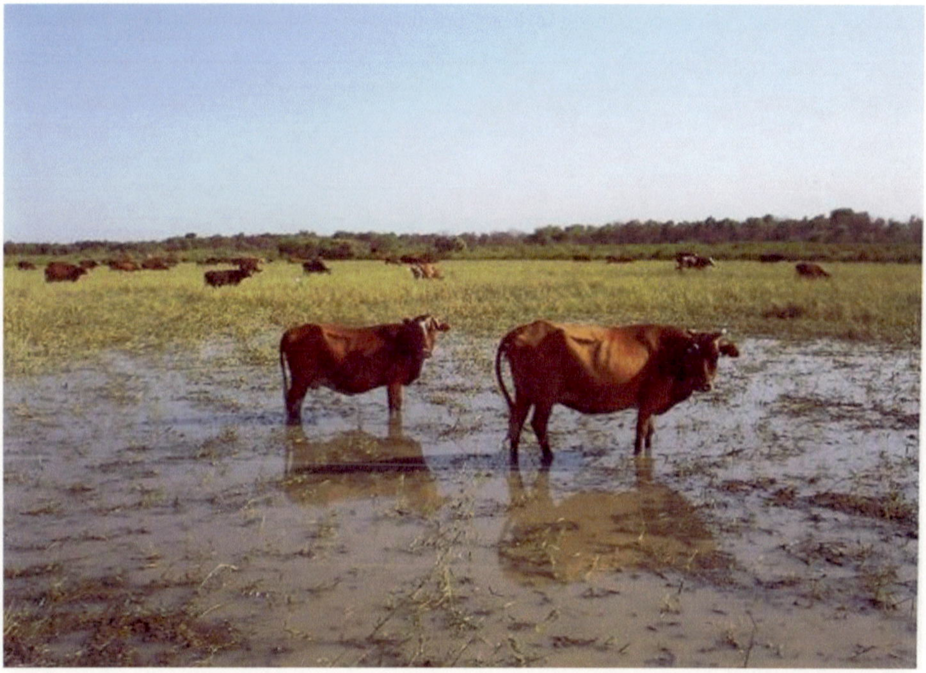

Figure 1.
*Foci of cercarioses (*Sch. turkestanicum*) in the territory of the republic of Karakalpakistan [25].*

serum can form. When scratched, the blisters break and produce small eroded areas, which then become covered with crust.

The boundary of the damaged areas depends on how deeply in water the person has been. If they only put their feet in water, the cercarie would penetrate the skin beneath the ankles, if they plunged waist-deep, the waist will be the upper boundary and so on. However, the cercariae usually do not penetrate the palms or soles.

The itching continues for one week or a little longer, depending on the sensitivity of the person's skin. The papules remain for about 6–7 days; then they disappear leaving red itching spots with crust in the centre. Later the crusts fall off, but these areas remain pigmented for some time.

The strong infection makes the organism sensitive to the disease, and subsequent infections cause allergic reactions.

S.A. Bear and M.V. Voronin (2007) indicate that the pathogenesis and morphology of cercarioses are determined by a number of factors, the most important of which are the following ones: (1) the mechanical damage of the skin when they penetrate it and migrate in it; (2) the toxic and sensitising effect the cercariae's metabolic and disintegration products cause; (3) the impact of the disintegration products from the tissues damaged by the larvae on the human organism. The degree to which these factors affect the organism depends on the number of the cercariae that have penetrated the skin, the number of penetrations, the species of the cercariae, their activity, their age and the state, in which the human organism is currently in, that is, the person's age, state of their skin, accompanying diseases, areas of penetration and so on. At the very moment of the penetration and within the first hours after it, the skin and mucous

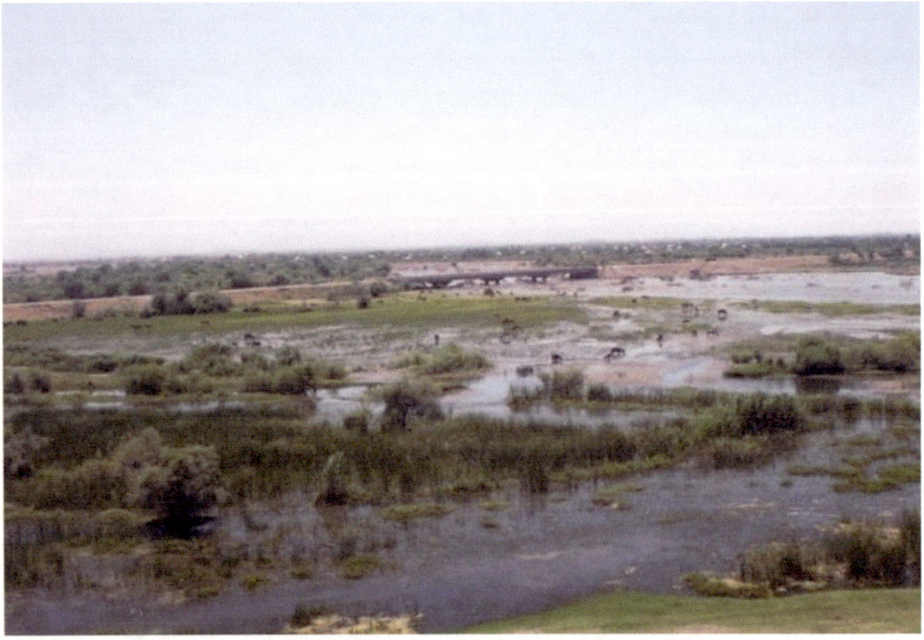

Figure 2.
*Foci of cercarioses (*Sch. turkestanicum*) in the territory of Tashkent Province [25].*

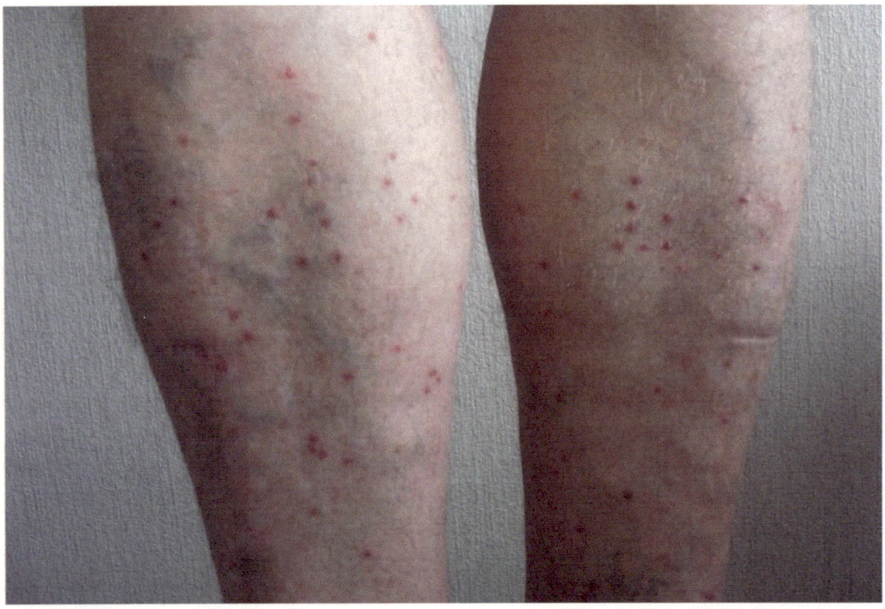

Figure 3.
Cercarioses caused by cercariae Sch. Turkestanicum *[25].*

membrane are damaged chemically and mechanically by the penetrating cercariae. Having attached to the skin with the help of the sucker, the cercariae can penetrate through the epidermis into the deeper layers of the skin within 5–10 minutes, using proteolytic enzymes emitted by the penetration glands. Large numbers of cercariae produce numerous cavities in the epidermis, as they penetrate through it.

Apart from the mechanical damage, the parasites damage it with the help of their enzymes, while the organism is sensitised by the metabolic and disintegrating products by the cercariae and the damaged human tissues and the tissues contain microflora, including the pathogenic. This is accompanied by the dilation and inflammation of the blood vessels of the superficial layers of the skin, their infiltration with its eosinophils and neutrophils, the oedema of the skin and the damage to its superficial layer. The damaged skin may have different forms (papules, petechial and popular skin rash, erythema, pigmented spots, granulomatous formations and others). Usually, they do not cause serious destructive changes in the tissues. The granulomae form around the cercariae that have died within the skin. The allergic reaction caused by the cercariae's alien proteins comes 5–6 hours later and is accompanied by strong itching, erythema and papules that appear on the skin in the places where the cercariae penetrated the skin.

The facts given above allow us to note two factors important from the epizootological and epidemiological aspects:

1. molluscs with cercariae found early in June can cause infection in specific hosts and humans (non-specific hosts);

2. the high rate of infection in molluscs and the emission of large numbers of mature cercariae in summer and early autumn can lead to a mass infection of humans in bodies of water and outbreaks of cercarioses in infection nidi.

The prevention of cercarioses includes personal hygiene and general preventive measures [5]. Sanitary education aimed to explain the ecology of the risk to be infected with cercariae of the trematode under study is the base of personal preventive measures and hygiene.

The complex of general preventive measures must aim at the reduction of the numbers of molluscs, the trematodes' intermediate hosts and at the diagnostic study of their definitive hosts. To prevent cercarioses effectively it is necessary to use all possible means of sanitary propaganda in order to explain to people the essence of the problem, the ecology and biology of the cercariae and the trematode's intermediate hosts and the ways to prevent the diseases.

Thus, cercarioses caused by *Sch. turkestanicum* in bodies of water in Uzbekistan and other countries require the most scrupulous attention from biologists and zoologists and cooperative actions from the veterinary and medical services.

Author details

Firuza D. Akramova[1], Djalaliddin A. Azimov[1], Ulugbek A. Shakarbaev[1] and Alisher A. Safarov[2*]

1 Institute of Zoology of the Academy of Sciences of the Republic of Uzbekistan, Tashkent, Uzbekistan

2 State Committee of Veterinary and Livestock Development of the Republic of Uzbekistan, Tashkent, Uzbekistan

*Address all correspondence to: safarov-alisher@mail.ru

References

[1] Azimov DA. The biology of Ornithobilharzia turkestanica in Uzbekistan. Report by the Academy of Sciences. 1969;7:52-53

[2] Kurochkin YV. Dermatitis of human caused by trematode cercariae in the volga delta. Всесоюзного общество гельминтов АН СССР. Moscow: Science; 1958. pp. 75-76

[3] Kurochkin YV. On dermatitis of human caused by trematode cercariae in the Volga delta. Helmintologia. 1959;**14**:225-229

[4] Horak P, Kolářova L, Adema CM. Biology of the Schistosoma genus Trichibilharzia. Advances in Parasitology. 2002;**52**:156-233

[5] Bear SA, Voronin MV. Cercarioses in Urban Ecosystems. Moscow: Nauka; 2007. p. 240

[6] Akramova FD, Azimov DA. The ecological and faunistic analysis of trematodes from the family Bilharziellidae Price, 1929. The Uzbek Biological Journal. 2005;**5**:47-52

[7] Akramova FD, Shakarboyev EB, Golovanov VI, Isakova DT, Azimov DA. The life cycle of trematode Dendritobilharzia loossi (Schistosomatida, Bilharziellidae), parasite of aquatic birds. The Bulletin of Zoology. 2007;**6**(41):511-520

[8] Akramova FD. Trematodes Bilharziellidae; their Origin and Evolution: A Doctoral Thesis. Tashkent: Institute of Zoology; 2011. p. 229

[9] Azimov DA, Akramova FD, Shakarbayev UA, Shakarboyev EB. Orientobildgarsii—Mammalian Trematodes. Tashkent: Fan; 2014. p. 224

[10] Chu GW. First report of the presence of a dermatitis-producing marine larval schistosomei Hawaii. Science. 1952;**115**:151-153

[11] Azimov DA, Arifjanov ZK. Research into the blood serum proteins of sheep infected experimentally with orientobilharziasis. The works of All-Russian Skrjabin Scientific Research Institute of Helmonthology. 1969;**15**:25-32

[12] Oda T. In: Morishita K et al., editors. Schistosome Dermatitis in Japan // Progress of Medical Parasitology in Japan. Vol. 5. Tokyo: Meguro Parasitological Museum; 1973. pp. 5-63

[13] Kumar V. Studies on snail hosts of Orientobilharzia turkestanicum (Skrjabin, 1913) Dutt et Srivastava, 1955 (Schistosomatidae: Trematoda) in India. Annales de la Société Belge de Médecine Tropicale. 1973;**53**(1):17-23

[14] Zakhryalov YN. On the methods of testing anti-orientobilharziasis medicines on rabbits. The questions of scientific research methods in the agriculture of Siberia and the Far East. 1972;**2**:150-152

[15] Zakhryalov YN. Orientobilharziaturkestanica (Skrjabin, 1913) Dutt and Srivastava, 1955 in the Far East: The abstract of a doctoral thesis. Alma-Ata. 1975:43

[16] Sahba Gholam HA, Malek EA. Dermatitis caused by cercariae of Orientobilharzia turkestanica in the Caspian Sea area of Iran. American Journal of Tropical Medicine and Hygiene. 1979;**28**(5):912-912

[17] Shakarboyev EB. The Ecological and Functional Interrelations of Orientobilharzia Turkestanica (Skrjabin, 1913) – Bos taurus Linnaeus, 1758 in the Parasite-Host System: A PhD Thesis in Biology. Tashkent; 1996. p. 134

[18] Shakarboyev EB. Trematodes of the Vertebrates of Uzbekistan (the Species Composition, Circulation Ways, Ecology Ad Biology): A Doctoral Thesis in Biology. Tashkent; 2009. p. 243

[19] Shakarboev EB, Akramova FZ, Golovanov VI, Azimov DA. Recommendations for the Prevention of Schistosomatosis in Livestock and Poultry. Tashkent; 2008. p. 27

[20] Kojabayev M. The Associative Infection with Trematodes in the Cattle (Bos taurus, Linnaeus, 1758) of the Aral Sea Area: A PhD Thesis. Tashkent; 2001. p. 98

[21] Amid A, Gohar S, Rosnami M. Dermination of definitive and intermediate hosts of cercarial dermatitis-producing agents in northern Iran. Archives of Iranian Medicine. 2006;**9**(1):11-15

[22] Wang CR, Pi BA, Song Z, Yu SJ, Zhang JM, Wang MY, et al. Investigation on the epidemic situation and the distribution feature of Orientobilharziasis ib cattle and sheep in Heilonjiang. Program in Veterinary Medicine. 2002;**23**:91-93

[23] Wang CR, Li L, Ni HB, Zhai YQ, Chen AH, Cheh J, et al. Orientobilharzia turcestanicum is a member of Schistosoma genus based on phylogenetic analysis using ribosomal DNA sequences. Experimental Parasitology. 2009;**121**:193-197

[24] Majoros G, Dan A, Erdelyi K. A natural focus of the blood fluke Orientobilharzia turkestanica (Skrjabin, 1913) (Trematoda: Schistosomatidae) in red deer (Cervus elaphus) in Hungery. Veterinary Parasitology. 2010;**170**(3-4):218-223

[25] Azimov DA, Akramova FD, Shakarboyev EB, Norqobilov BT, Shakarbayev UA, Sayitqulov BS. Schistosomiasis of Animals. Tashkent: Fan; 2019. p. 320

Chapter 10

Conclusion

Djalaliddin A. Azimov

The problem of schistosomiasis caused by *Sch. turkestanicum* is many-sided. It combines general biological, veterinary, medical, economic and social questions and their interrelations. Data on the pathogenic agents of schistosomiasis have been available since the nineteenth century. Their evolution, as that of all schistosomatides, is peculiar and mysterious [1–3]. The knowledge of *Sch. turkestanicum* causing infectious diseases in animals and cercarioses in humans has been accumulated for a long time. Numerous studies conducted in many countries of Asia and Europe have shown that populations of *Sch. turkestanicum* are quite widespread among synanthropic and wild mammals, while diseases caused by them are transregional.

Schistosomiasis of animals occurs in acute and chronic forms. The parasitising of *Sch. turkestanicum* in the lumina of blood vessels and their feeding on blood and metabolic products predetermine the entire symptomatic complex of the disease.

Together with mature parasites, the laid eggs play a significant role in the pathogenesis of schistosomiasis. The eggs laid by female trematodes in the vessels of inner organs cause serious reactions in the tissues of the liver, spleen and intestinal tract. Migrating eggs cause damage to the integrity of vessels of organs and tissues, which was confirmed by histological studies [2, 4–7]. Quite serious reactive changes were recorded in the liver and submucous layer of the thin intestine. Limited nodes emerging as a result of egg accumulation are recorded everywhere. There are signs of degeneration in strongly infected animals, diarrhoea characterised by a mixture of blood and exhaustion of animals. In general, this disease adversely affects the growth, development, productivity and reproduction in cattle.

Our long-term studies carried out in the biogeocenoses of Uzbekistan enabled us to make a clear picture of the role of *Sch. turkestanicum* in the pathology of animals and the nature of formation of individual concentrations and current distribution in different regions and find answers for many questions.

This book is the first monograph in the world-generalising data on the morphology and biology of all development stages, and ecological peculiarities and infection of intermediate and definitive hosts. Trematodes are highly pathogenic for synanthropic and wild mammals, which enables to solve a number of questions of parasite-host interrelations.

In this book, significant attention is paid to the distribution of schistosomiasis of animals and cercariosis of human in Asian and European countries. The work considers the methods of diagnosis, treatment and prevention of infection on the basis of modern understanding. A wide range of theoretical and practical problems solved using the example of *Sch. turkestanicum* is predetermined by a high interest to this infection in the late twentieth and early twenty-first centuries. This is confirmed by the results of the recent studies, including those in the sphere of molecular biology of *Sch. turkestanicum* [8–13].

Available ecological data on this *Schistosoma* suggest a good level of knowledge of *Sch. turkestanicum* and its confinement to the Asian region. However, this opinion is not quite right. A subspecies of *Sch. turkestanicum* was recorded in sheep in Turkey and quite recently in deer in Hungary [13]. A closer study may help find this trematode in other countries too, where biological preconditions are suitable for the development and distribution of this parasite.

This book does not aim to cover fully and comprehensively all schistosomiasis-related problems. We had a plainer goal, which was to generalise the results of the research into this trematode from the biological and economic aspects from the moment of its discovery in 1913 to the present day (2020).

We believe that the total amount of generalised materials serves as a reliable methodological basis for further studies on all problems relating to schistosomiasis of animals and cercariosis of human in certain regions of the world, first and foremost in Asian and European countries.

Thus, the strategy of schistosomiasis should aim at the decrease of the infection control through control of the size of mollusc populations; dehelminthisation of animals, the sources of infection; creation of new and more effective medicines; a strict adherence to veterinary and sanitary norms at farms and in the wild.

Author details

Djalaliddin A. Azimov
Institute of Zoology of the Academy of Sciences of the Republic of Uzbekistan, Tashkent, Uzbekistan

*Address all correspondence to: safarov-alisher@mail.ru

References

[1] Azimov DA, Shakarboyev EB, Akramova FD, Shakarbayev UA. Orientobilgartsioz: Diagnostika and Profilaktika (handout). Tashkent: Institute of Zoology; 2010. p. 8

[2] Azimov DA, Akramova FD, Shakarbayev UA, Shakarboyev EB. Orientobildgarsii—Mammalian Trematodes. Tashkent: Fan; 2014. p. 224

[3] Azimov DA, Akramova FD, Shakarboyev EB, Norqobilov BT, Shakarbayev UA, Sayitqulov BS. Schistosomiasis of Animals. Tashkent: Fan; 2019. p. 320

[4] Azimov DA, Nurmukhamedov KN. Orientobilharziasis in ruminants. The Agriculture of Uzbekistan. 1967;7:56

[5] Azimov DA, Nurmukhamedov KN. New data on the biology of trematode Orientobilharzia turkestanica (Schistosomatidae). The Zoological Magazine. 1968;**10**:1471-1478

[6] Azimov DA, Nurmukhamedov KN. The pathomorphology of orientobilharziasis of sheep and goats. The collection of works on helminthology dedicated to the 90th anniversary of K.I. Skrjabin. Moscow; 1971. pp. 5-11

[7] Lavrov LI, Vsevolodov BP. Materials on the pathomorphology of orientobilharziasis of cattle. Helminths and helminthiases of animals of Kazakhstan. Works by the Institute of Zoology under the Academy of Sciences of the Republic of Kazakhstan. 1967;**27**:156-168

[8] Snyder SD, Loker ES. Evolutionary relationships among the Schistosomatidae (Platyhelminthes: Digenea) and an Asian origin for Schistosoma. Parasitology. 2000;**86**:283-288

[9] Lockyer AE, Olson PD, Littlewood DTJ. Utility of complete large and small subunit rRNA genes in resolving the phylogeny of the Platyhelminthes: Implications and review of the cercomer theory. Biologikal Journal of the Linnean Society. 2003;**78**:155-173

[10] Li L, Yu LY, Zhu XQ, Wang CR, Zhai YQ, Zhao JP. Orientobilharzia turkestanicum is grouped within African schistosomes based on phylogenetic analyses using sequences of mitochondrial genes. Parasitology Research. 2008;**102**:939-943

[11] Qiu JH, Li L, Wang CR, Chen J, Chen AH, Zhai YQ. ITS and 28S rDNA-LSU sequence analysis of Orientobilharzia turkestanicum from bovine and caprine hosts. Chinese Journal of Parasitology. 2008;**26**(3):183

[12] Wang CR, Li L, Ni HB, Zhai YQ, Chen AH, Cheh J, et al. Orientobilharzia turcestanicum is a member of Schistosoma genus based on phylogenetic analysis using ribosomal DNA sequences. Experimental Parasitology. 2009;**121**:193-197

[13] Majoros G, Dán A, Erdélyi K. A natural focus of the blood fluke *Orientobilharzia turkestanica* (Skrjabin, 1913) (Trematoda: Schistosomatidae) in red deer (*Cervus elaphus*) in Hungery. Veterinary Parasitology. 2010;**170**(3-4):218-223